I0018391

Information and IT for Dentistry: a

Professor Alan Gillies MA PhD FBCS CITP
Professor of Information Management
Lancashire School of Health and Postgraduate Medicine
PRESTON, PR1 2HE, Lancashire, UK

ISBN: 978-1-84753-069-1

This book was written to celebrate the launch of undergraduate dental education at the University of Central Lancashire in 2007

Preface

This book has been designed to help dentists to establish and maintain information systems that are necessary for effective working. It will consider the context of dentists in the UK, USA and Canada.

It tries to do at least six impossible things:

Six (almost!) impossible things

1. Talk about information in an interesting way.

2. Show how information can actually be useful.

3. Explain how to get you to love your computer.

4. Make SNODENT Codes interesting.

5. Help practices to share meaningful information.

6. Make you smile while reading a book about information.

It includes references to incredibly unhip comedy series such as 'The Hitch Hiker's Guide to the Galaxy' (such as why not round off this chapter by breakfast at Milliways, the Restaurant at the End of the Universe?).

The book assumes that you the reader are based in, or work with, a dental practice. Each chapter includes exercises that generally require you to have access to a dental practice.

There is a web site associated with this book. While it will be advantageous to have access to this, the book is designed to be largely accessible without Web access.

The book was fun to write. I hope it's fun to read.

Alan Gillies

January 2007

How to use the book

The book is organised into a series of chapters. Broadly speaking, it is probably best if you read them in order. However, you may well find some material surplus to requirements.

There are a number of common elements that recur throughout the book. Many of these have icons to help you spot them:

 Exercises

Exercises generally occur at the end of chapters. They are designed to be carried out either by an individual or a group. They have a distinct output, generally in the form of a table. Model answers are given at the end of the book, but on the understanding that these are model answers. As most of the exercises relate to the readers' own experience, they may well have different detailed answers to the model answers given. The purpose of the model answers is to give an indication of the style of answer rather than the actual content.

 Think Box

Before we leave this chapter think about the following questions:

Think Boxes are designed to explore issues raised in the preceding chapters and exercises. They are designed for discussion, and would really benefit from the chance to discuss the answers with colleagues, either in a group situation or in a series of one-to-one encounters.

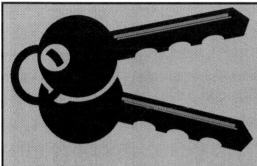

Key points from this chapter

Key points are given at the end of each chapter to reinforce the key learning outcomes. They should not be used as a short cut, but rather as a check on knowledge gained. By the time you have completed the exercise, thought about the Think Box, and reinforced key points, you should be ready to move on to the next chapter.

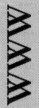

Web link

This is a World Wide Web link. It refers to resources accessible via the associated Web pages which may be found at:

http://www.IT4dentists.com

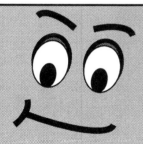

Smile!

These are anecdotes to make you smile. If the smile looks a bit lopsided, you may understand when you read the accompanying text!

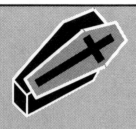

Zombie warning

The concept of the intellectual zombie was introduced by Professor Bob Evans of British Colombia in Canada.

An intellectual zombie is an idea that refuses to die in spite of all the evidence to the contrary

Points in a numbered list

You will find numbered lists throughout the text to emphasise material within the text.

Other key passages are highlighted in tables such as this.

Finally, don't forget the list of abbreviations and explanation of terms used in the Appendix. It contains explanation of a range of technical terms.

Table of Contents

List of Figures

List of Tables

Chapter 1 Why do we need information?

Many dentists use computers to manage their business. At the same time, you may not be using your computers to the best effect in your clinical practice.

Why should we want better information?

My job is information. It's what I do. But if you are a dentist, or a dental nurse, or a dental practice manager, then your job is dentistry, and that's what you do. So why do you need better information?

I suggest that there are four reasons why you might wish to have better information:

Four reasons why you might want better information

1. To make more money

2. To save money

3. To provide better care for your patients

4. To reduce the risk of doing harm to your patients

Table 1 Four reasons why you might want better information

If someone wants you to spend money or time in order to get better information, then ask them whether it will help you achieve any of these and if so, how?

In reality, in some cases, you can achieve more than one benefit. For example,

- If you reduce the chance of an adverse event, thereby reducing the risk of doing harm to your patients, you should be a better risk for your insurance company, and that should save you money.

- Alternatively, if you use information to track your patients better, then you should recall them more often and reliably. This should be good for your patients' oral health. Assuming that your remuneration is linked to your level of activity, then, it should also increase your income.

In the same way, the division between management and clinical activity may not be so clear cut. There is a whole area of activity which may be characterised as "clinical management". Better information and the use of associated technology to process it can lead to the systemisation of practice, and improvements in patients' health and dentists' income.

In order to see how this may apply to you, then try this first exercise:

☑ Exercise 1

To get you thinking about information make a list of all the pieces of information using the categories listed in the table below.

Patient name and address details	Patient dental details
Financial information	**Other information**

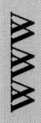

Web Link

All the exercises are available from the web site as templates.

They are available for download as either Acrobat (.pdf) files for printing and then filling in by hand, or Rich Text Files for processing on your PC

Dentists, in common with other health care professionals have always used information. The classical information system in dental care has been paper-based, with paper forms stored in envelopes. This may not seem very sexy as information systems go, but it served dentists quite well for many decades

Before we move on, let's think about this classical information system on which dentists have depended for so long for their clinical information.

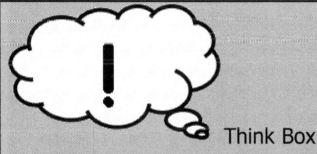

Think Box

1.   What are the advantages of the paper-based information system?

2.   What are the disadvantages?

3.   What are the specific things that you want to do that you can't do with a paper-based system?

4.   Are there risks that your patients face if you leave your information in a paper-based system?

Any replacement system must do better than this. In spite of the promise of new technology, many dental practices still depend on their old paper-based systems for much of their work. This may be because they still see the purpose of records as the traditional aide-memoire for the dental practitioner, and paper records are very good for this purpose.

In 2003, in a survey of English dental practices found nearly a quarter of practices still were not using computers at all[1].

Of those not using computers, over half (56%) stated that they didn't believe they were not currently necessary. Around one quarter cited staff reluctance (24%), whilst slightly less said that the systems were too expensive (19%). Only 45% had Internet and Email access at this time.

In spite of dentistry in the UK still being part of the National Health Service, and the National Programme for IT spending billions to join up the entire Service, plans to connect dentistry to the rest of the system via the N3 network are still in the early stages and lag well behind the connection rates in almost every other section of the health care system.

However, technology is not an end in itself, it is a means to deliver the information that is needed to support the management and care of dental patients. The purpose of this handbook is to help you set up good systems to provide your practice with high quality information. Only a small part of this task is about computers, so only a small part of this book is about them. First, we must identify the information that we need.

---

[1] *J. H. John, D. Thomas and D. Richards (2003) Questionnaire survey on the use of computerisation in dental practices across the Thames Valley region, British Dental Journal, 195, 585–590.*

Key points from this chapter

Information is a key part of all parts of health care and dentistry is no exception.

You should want better information not for its own sake but in order to deliver specific benefits for you and your patients

Dental practitioners have always kept records and used information to manage the care of their patients

Paper-based information systems do have advantages as an aide memoire: they are flexible, require no special skills to use and no expensive equipment to store and handle them

Paper-based systems impose limitations on the management of care, and computer-based systems can offer significant advantages

Chapter 2 What information do we need?

In any situation, the information needed is determined by the tasks that we are required to carry out.

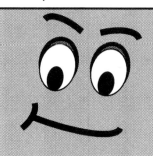

Smile!

Information needs should be determined by organisational or user objectives (and not the other way around!)

However, as an esteemed colleague has observed frequently:

"Perfectly logical, never happen here!"

Traditionally, dentists have collected information for two key purposes:

- As an aide memoire: to make a record of care for the next time that the patient visits.

- To obtain payment for services rendered from either the patient, an insurance company, dental plan provider or a public health care system.

However, even paper records have been used for other purposes:

Traditional purposes for which information is used

In addition to the two main purposes:

1. As an aide memoire: to make a record of care for the next time that the patient visits.

2. To obtain payment for services rendered from either the patient, an insurance company, dental plan provider or a public health care system.

Dentists have used paper records to

3. carry out retrospective audit and research

4. justify and defend their actions in the event of complaints or problems

5. communicate the nature of, and reasons for, treatment to patients

Table 2 Traditional purposes for which information is used

Think Box

1. For what other uses have you historically collected information?
2. What are the disadvantages of using paper–based records for these?

The reality is that the modern environment in which dentistry is operating needs more and better information for a wider range of purposes, including:

Purposes for which more and better information is needed

1. Matching supply and demand for dental services
2. Increased emphasis on health promotion
3. Clinical governance
4. Greater emphasis on patient choice based on informed consent
5. Cost control

Table 3 Purposes for which more and better information is needed

Ha! Many of you will home in on the last purpose and say that this is the real reason. In many ways you would be right. In all aspects of health care, people are concerned about the rate at which costs are rising.

Here is the percentage of the Gross Domestic Product spent on health care by the US, Canada and the UK every five years since 1988, as measured by the OECD.

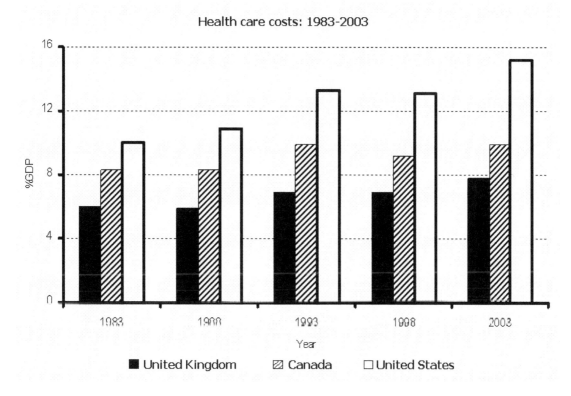

Figure 1 Rising health care costs in the UK, Canada and the USA (Source:OECD)

Whether you are an individual patient, insurance company, or Government, these are fairly scary figures if you are paying for care. Of course, those being paid may well not have seen the benefit as costs rise in terms of materials, indemnity insurance and other factors.

This has led to an environment characterised by the following characteristics:

- Constant health care reform in both the public and private sector. In dentistry in the UK, this has the added dimension of threatening to destroy the balance between public and private dentistry. If too much reform and cost control is introduced in the public sector, then dentists will simply withdraw into the private sector.

- Pressure for efficiency savings, and IT is heralded as a major source of such savings (see, for example, the Wanless Reports in the UK[2],[3], or the Romanow

---

[2] *Wanless, D Securing Our Future Health: Taking a Long-Term View, Report for HM Treasury, April 2002, HMSO, London.*

[3] *Wanless D Securing Good Health for the Whole Population, Report for HM Treasury, February 2004, HMSO, London.*

commission in Canada[4]). Whilst they may appear to have little direct to say about dentistry, they say a great deal about the environment in which dentistry operates. Similarly, whilst they speak primarily of the public system , the same pressures apply in the private sector, and may bite even more rapidly there

Web Link

Both these reports are available to download from the web site accompanying the book.

- Emphasis upon health not disease and prevention rather than cure. Health and prevention are double winners: they can achieve better care whilst saving money. This is irresistible for any Government, insurance company, or even private individual. However, prevention and health promotion are expensive in terms of the demands that they place upon information and the associated technology.

At its simplest, we need to know about our patients and about the activities undertaken to keep them healthy or restore them to health when they are ill. This means we have to keep information about patients and about procedures. In the previous chapter we identified two types of patient information: basic information about the patient known as demographic data, and information about their medical history. Information about procedures was considered under two headings: financial and other. However, in these post-market days, we should perhaps simply refer to activity data, and consider information about the quantity and quality of activity.

For our second exercise, we can use a modified version of the table in Exercise 1 to consider both the information requirements and the tasks that they support.

To complete the exercise, identify both the information and the tasks for which it is needed. The bottom row has changed slightly asking you to consider performance management, both from the point of quantity, often reflected in remuneration, and quality, which is not.

---

[4] *Romanow, R Building on Values: The Future of Health Care in Canada, Final report of the Commission on the future of health care in Canada, ISBN 0-662-330343-9*

☑ Exercise 2

To establish what information we might need make a list of all the pieces of information using the categories listed in the table below.

Patient demographics		Patient dental details	
Information	**Tasks**	**Information**	**Tasks**
How many activities?		**How good is the activity?**	
Information	**Tasks**	**Information**	**Tasks**

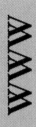

Web Link

Don't forget, all the exercises are available from the web site as templates.

They are available for download as either Acrobat (.pdf) files for printing and then filling in by hand, or Rich Text Files for processing on your PC.

I shan't mention this again, lest you get bored of hearing about this.

Fortunately, we do not have to work out for ourselves, the information and functions that we need from our systems. Other clever people have done that for us.

For example, in the USA, there are a range of standards and technical guides approved by the American National Standards Association and the American Dental Association to define what a dental information system should be, as shown in Table 4. We may consider just one of these in more detail, the first specification defining the structure and content of an electric health record, shown in Table 5.

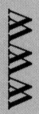

Web Link

These standards are available to download from the web, but the detailed standards are subject to a significant charge.

The English NHS documents are available free of charge and linked from the website

- ADA Specification No. 1004: Computer Software Performance for Dental Practice Software

- ANSI/ADA Specification No. 1000: Standard Clinical Data Architecture for the Structure and Content of an Electric Health Record

- ANSI/ADA Specification No. 1001: Guidelines for the Design of Educational Software

- ADA Technical Report No. 1006 for Infection Control for Dental Information Systems

- ADA Technical Report No. 1010 for Accounting Performance for Dental Information Systems

- ADA Technical Report No. 1012 for Hardware Recommendations for Dental Information Systems

- ADA Technical Report No. 1016 for Electronic Signature Applications in Dentistry

- ADA Technical Report No. 1017 for Administrative Procedures and their application in Dentistry

- ADA Technical Report No. 1018: Technical Security Mechanisms and Their Application to Dentistry

- ADA Technical Report No. 1019 for Technical Security Services and Application to Dentistry

- ADA Technical Report No. 1020: Physical Safeguards and Applications to Dentistry

- ADA Technical Report No. 1021:Data Integrity, Redundancy, Storage and Accessibility

- ADA Technical Report No. 1023: Implementation Requirements for DICOM in Dentistry

- ADA Technical Report No. 1027: Implementation Guide for ANSI/ADA Specification No. 1000

- ADA Technical Report No. 1029 for Digital Photography

- ADA Technical Report No. 1031 for internet Security Issues for Dental Information Systems

Table 4: ADA Standards Committee on Dental Informatics Standards and technical guides

---

ANSI/ADA Specification No. 1000: Standard Clinical Data Architecture for the Structure and Content of an Electric Health Record

On February 2, 2001, the ANSI/ADA 1000 for the Standard Clinical Data Architecture for the Structure and Content of an Electronic Health Record was approved by as an American National Standard. The standard includes the following parts:

Part 1000.0 Introduction, Model Architecture, and Specification Framework
Part 1000.1 Individual Identification
Part 1000.2 Codes and Nomenclature
Part 1000.3 Individual Characteristics
Part 1000.4 Population Characteristics
Part 1000.5 Organization
Part 1000.6 Location
Part 1000.7 Communication
Part 1000.8 Health Care Event
Part 1000.9 Health Care Materiel
Part 1000.10 Health Services
Part 1000.11 Health Service Resources
Part 1000.12 Population Health Facts
Part 1000.13 Patient Health Facts
Part 1000.14 Health Condition Diagnosis
Part 1000.15 Patient Service Plan
Part 1000.16 Patient Health Service
Part 1000.17 Clinical Investigation
Part 1000.18 Comments Subject Area

Table 5: ANSI/ADA Specification No. 1000

In the UK, public dentistry falls under the NHS, and also under the remit of the National Programme for IT if you are based in England. In 2002, the document *An Information Technology Strategy for NHS Dentistry in the 21st Century*[5] promised:

1.2   Delivering *21st Century IT Support for the NHS* outlines a vision for the future of information in the NHS. The priorities and challenges for NHS dentistry fit within this NHS-wide strategic approach to IT.

1.3   The overriding theme of Options for Change (OfC) is the re-integration of dentistry within the NHS and for dental records to become more connected with mainstream NHS IT.

1.4   OfC requires the development and application of a standard oral health assessment and clinical pathways for dentistry, which will need to be applied

---

[5] *An Information Technology Strategy for NHS Dentistry in the 21st Century, October 2002, HMSO, London*

---

consistently across the NHS. These will all need the support of an integrated IT strategy.

1.5　　Electronic records including digitised radiographs will need to be transferable between dentists and other organisations

1.6　　To achieve this vision, there will need to be a substantial investment in education, training and change management for dental practice

In spite of this, the vision of a dental service connected to itself and to the rest of the health care system remains elusive.

Think Box

Before we leave this chapter think about the following question:

In this chapter, we introduced the idea of a joined up vision of information systems supporting joined up dental and other health care, drawing on information from dental practice systems. What changes could you make to the information and the way that it is stored to reduce the barriers identified in Exercise 3?

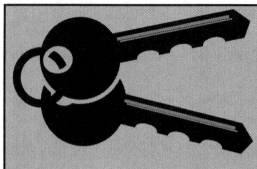

Key points from this chapter

The information needed by dentists is determined by the tasks that dentists are required to carry out.

In the USA, the American Dental Association has published details standards defining what should be in a dental information system

In England, public dentistry is covered within the scope of the NHS National Programme for IT, but progress is slow towards linking dentists up to the national infrastructure

☑ Exercise 3

The above vision depends on dental practices sharing access to the information contained in their practice systems. What barriers are there to this?

Technical barriers	
Legal barriers	
Human barriers	

Chapter 3 You really mean computers, don't you?

So far we have managed to avoid the c******* word. (Well almost, we've mentioned it a few times, in fact). Maybe you're getting cross because you thought this book was going to be about computers and you thought I was joking in Chapter 1 (what do you mean you didn't read it because it was only an introduction?). OK, for any techies among you here goes…a chapter on computers!

The trouble with computers in the UK NHS is too often they have been like elephants

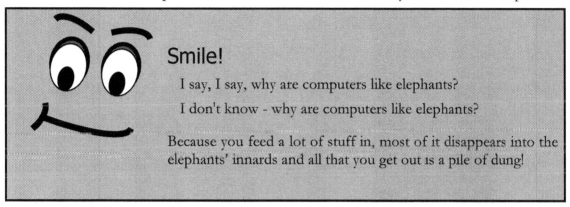

Smile!

I say, I say, why are computers like elephants?

I don't know - why are computers like elephants?

Because you feed a lot of stuff in, most of it disappears into the elephants' innards and all that you get out is a pile of dung!

The history of the NHS and IT is not a happy one. Ask the Secretary of State…

'Up to now the use of IT in the NHS has not been a success story. Far from it. Lots of money has been wasted. Some important data has not been collected and used. Other data has been collected but not used…'

Table 6 Frank Dobson, in the Foreword to Information for Health (1998).

Add to this, the traditional feeling that dentistry is on the fringes of the NHS and the chances of using technology to join dentists up to the rest of the health service seem slim.

Here's my list of some of the reasons why IT hasn't been a success.

Ten reasons why IT hasn't been a success in public dentistry such as within the English NHS

1 IT has been technology-driven not information-driven.

2 Too much has been spent on technology instead of training.

3 Technology has been seen as an end in itself.

4 Many failures have been due to basic project management lessons.

5 NHS IT staff are poorly paid in comparison with the private sector.

6 The agenda has been driven by management issues, not clinicians.

7 The suppliers have not been regulated effectively.

8 GP systems are incompatible with each other.

9 The market system discouraged collaboration.

10 Codes are incomprehensible and have been badly implemented

Table 7 Ten reasons why IT hasn't been a success in public dentistry such as within the English NHS

However, it really doesn't have to be like this. Computers can actually make life easier (no, honestly, I mean it!). You do however need to do things a bit differently.

To get you started, there are at least ten good things you can do to help improve things. Please note that buying a new computer doesn't figure in my top ten, but I guess if you don't have one at all, maybe it should!

Ten ways to improve the chances of success with IT!

1. Start by considering information needs, not technology.
2. Invest heavily in training for clinical staff as well as admin staff.
3. Involve clinicians in all IT decisions.
4. Technology is a means to an end.
5. Use proper project management techniques.
6. Use the best IT support you can.
7. Ensure that the IT solution delivers better patient care and clinical benefits.
8. Ensure that the suppliers deliver what's promised.
9. Adopt recommended solutions across the Primary Care Trust to minimise compatibility problems with other dentists and clinicians
10. Agree a coding policy, with other stakeholders which covers all aspects of clinical practice as well as management activity

Table 8 Ten ways to improve the chances of success with IT!

These positive principles will guide the rest of the book. Computers can actually be a help. However, state-of-the-art technology is not a critical success factor. I have seen good information systems running on primitive technology but highly tailored to the needs of their practice, and I have seen state of the art technology producing rubbish.

Think Box

Before we leave this chapter think about the following question:

The Secretary of State said 'Some important data has not been collected and used. Other data has been collected but not used...' What examples can you give from your own work of:

    a) important data which has not been collected?

    b) other data that has been collected but not used?

If you try to introduce a new information system into a less than organised dental practice, it will make things worse, not better. I have never seen ANY evidence ANYWHERE that introducing technology into a disorganised practice helps sort things out. What it can do is provide the impetus for human beings to sort things out. If this can be achieved first, then the system can help make things better.

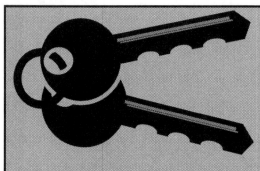

Key points from this chapter

The history of the NHS and IT is not a happy one.

There are at least 10 reasons for this

Computers can actually be a help.

State of the art technology is not a critical success factor

There are good information systems based around limited technology, and bad information systems based around advanced technology

Before any decisions are made about acquiring computer hardware and software, it is essential that the human and information systems are clearly established.

 Exercise 4

Use the table opposite to assess the digestive habits of your ~~elephant~~ computer system. Delete any information that you don't collect from the left-hand column and any from the right that doesn't come out again by sorting or searching

Information in	Information able to searched for or sorted by
Name of practice	Name of practice
ID number of practice	ID number of practice
Address(es) of surgery	Address(es) of surgery
Telephone and fax numbers	Telephone and fax numbers
Dentist's Name	Dentist's Name
Dentist's professional ID number	Dentist's professional ID number
Dental Nurse's Name	Dental Nurse's Name
Dental Nurse's professional ID number	Dental Nurse's professional ID number
Patient title	Patient title
Patient Surname	Patient Surname
Patient Forenames	Patient Forenames
Patient identifier	Patient identifier
Date of Birth	Date of Birth
Sex	Sex
Marital status	Marital status
Payment status (Full cost/Insured with co-payment/Fully insured/Public with co-payment/Exempt)	Payment status (Full cost/Insured with co-payment/Fully insured/Public with co-payment/Exempt)
Payment history	Payment history
Registered home address	Registered home address
Previous or alternative address	Previous or alternative address
Telephone contact number	Telephone contact number
Postcode	Postcode
Responsible health authority	Responsible health authority
General Practitioner/Family Physician	General Practitioner/Family Physician
Allergies	Allergies
Date and time of consultation	Date and time of consultation
Location of consultation	Location of consultation
Medical, family and social history	Medical, family and social history
Symptoms, signs and investigations	Symptoms, signs and investigations
Treatments	Treatments
Diagnoses, sensitivities and problems	Diagnoses, sensitivities and problems
Medical prescriptions	Medical prescriptions
Interactions and contraindications	Interactions and contraindications
Doses	Doses

Chapter 4 Why you need those horrible computers

Ah! You knew we'd get back to computers before too long, didn't you? We need computers because our paper-based systems simply cannot provide adequate information to support the information needs of a large modern dental practice let alone support shared information with the rest of the health community.

However, computers are simply a means to an end to deliver the information system we need. On their own, they cannot solve our problems. If you don't know how to get from London to Manchester, then having a fast car is as likely to take you away from Manchester as towards it.

Worse, if you set off in the wrong direction, the faster the car, the further away it will take you in a given period of time. Computers are fast cars compared with paper-based systems which are more like push bikes, but you can still head off hurtling towards the English Channel, if you don't know where you're going.

The purpose of this chapter is to understand better what computers can and cannot do, so that we can use them appropriately and effectively to achieve the goals of better dental care and practice management.

Let's first consider what computers are good at.

Ten things computers are good at

1. Storing information

2. Sorting information

3. Finding information

4. Working quickly

5. Doing what they are told

6. Talking to other computers

7. Passing on information to other computers quickly

8. Adding up and doing other sums

9. Producing pretty graphs from numbers

10. Sitting there and not getting impatient whilst waiting for the next instruction

---

Table 9 Ten things computers are good at

But equally, there are things that computers are bad at. Ten of these are listed below. The best way to think about this is to consider the computer as a member of your team, with particular strengths and weaknesses. As in any team situation good practice requires that you play to the computer's strengths and compensate for its weaknesses. Very often, problems are caused by people's false expectations of their computer systems.

Ten things computer are bad at

1. Being intelligent, computers are stupid
2. Computers do what you say, not what you want
3. Using judgement
4. Communicating with people
5. Applying contextual information
6. Working with fuzzy data, eg diagnoses
7. Remembering when power is switched off
8. Working the way people work
9. Telling when people are lying
10. Using common sense, they don't have any!

Table 10 Ten things computers are bad at

You always knew about the computer's limitations, didn't you? They can't help it, it's just the way they are made. Think of them as a member of your team. In any team situation, you analyse each member's strengths and weaknesses and utilise their strengths and avoid exacerbating their weaknesses. Treat the computer as a member of the team. Understand the strengths and weaknesses of your computer and play to its strengths.

Computers treat information very literally. To you, if the patient complains of toothache, you would likely look in the patients mouth. A computer wouldn't know where to look. Everything that you want the computer to know it has to be told.

For example, if you told the computer any of the following things shown in Table 11. It wouldn't even see a problem.

Five things a computer wouldn't know were wrong

1. the patient is –70 years old

2. the patient is 700 years old

3. the patient is older than his parents

4. the patient was born tomorrow

5. the patient is male and female

Table 11 Five things a computer wouldn't know were wrong

The computer will only query these statements if given a specific instruction so to do. Computers work best when information is precise and unambiguous. The problem is, that in healthcare, information rarely is.

Why bother? What's in it for you as a dentist?

- Dental office computer systems should be compatible with those of the hospitals and plans they conduct business with. Referral inquiries should be handled easily.

- Vendors should be able to supply low-cost software solutions to physicians/dentists who support standards-based EDI. Costs associated with mailing, faxing, and telephoning may decrease.

- Administrative tasks can be accomplished electronically. Dentists may have more time to devote to direct care.

- Dentists should have a more complete data set of the patient they are treating, enabling better care. More efficient systems may give dentists more time to spend with patients and performing clinical work.

Source: American Dental Association

Table 12 Why bother? What's in it for you as a dentist?

Why Bother? What's in it for your patients?

- Patients seeking information on enrolment status or health care benefits may be given more accurate, complete and easier-to-understand information.

- Cost savings to providers and plans may translate into less costly health care for consumers. Premiums and charges may be lowered.

- Patients may save postage and telephone costs incurred in claims follow-up.

- Patients should have the ability to see what is contained in their medical records. The infrastructure should be in place for patients to see who has accessed their medical records. Patient records should be adequately protected through organizational policies and technical security controls.

- Visits to dentists and other health care providers may be shorter without the burden of filling out forms.

- Consumer correspondence with insurers about problems with claims may be reduced.

Source: American Dental Association

Table 13 Why bother? What's in it for your patients?

In the next chapter, we shall see the major implication of using computers. In order to make effective use of computers, it is essential to represent information in a computer-friendly form. Unfortunately, this is not a people- friendly form. We must bite the bullet and look at structuring information for computers.

☑ Exercise 5

In this exercise, we want to look at the implications of the strengths and weaknesses of computers for their use in dental practice.

In the following table, think of an instance and the implication where each strength and weakness affects the management and delivery of healthcare within your own practice. One example is done to help you.

		Instance	Implication
Strength	Storing information Sorting information Finding information Working quickly Doing what they are told Talking to other computers Passing on information to other computers quickly Adding up and doing other sums Producing pretty graphs from numbers Sitting there and not getting impatient while waiting for the next instruction	Consultation	Can find patient record
Weakness	Not being intelligent Computers do what you say, not what you want They don't use judgement Bad at communicating with people Applying contextual information Working with fuzzy data, eg diagnoses Remembering when power is switched off Working the way people work Telling when people are lying Using common sense, they don't have any!		

Think Box

Before we leave this chapter think about the following questions:

Before we leave this chapter think about the following question:

Think about current computer systems in dental practices. What are the major barriers to making better use of information. How may they be dismantled?

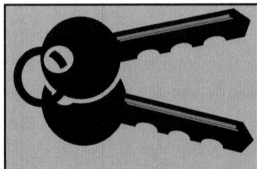

Key points from this chapter

Paper-based systems simply cannot provide adequate information to support the information needs of an integrated health care system.

Computers are simply a means to an end to deliver the information system we need.

On their own, computers cannot solve our problems

Computers have very particular strengths

Computers have very particular weaknesses

It is necessary to understand the strengths and weaknesses of computers in order to play to their strengths.

Chapter 5 Why you need those even more horrible codes

In the overall scale of things, dental or drug codes are not attractive objects. They do not have ascetic beauty, mathematical elegance or even basic comprehensibility.

It is therefore unfortunate that coding schema are probably the second most important thing to get right about your information solution (the first being the people side of things). So the first job must be to explain why coding is important and which codes are important to dentistry. It is perhaps too much to hope that you should ever come to love such codes, and frankly if you do, then the best advice is either to get a life or seek professional counselling.

People use natural language to communicate and to describe things. It has the advantage of being known to everyone, very flexible, able to express shades of opinion and fuzziness. However, from the computer's point of view it is complex, inconsistent and requires a great deal of contextual information to interpret ambiguities. As we have seen, computers can process information quickly, but only if it is clear and unambiguous.

Just as human language has evolved to meet our information processing needs, so systems have evolved to meet the information processing needs of computers. Coding systems meet a need to describe the world of healthcare in concise and unambiguous ways.

The first major coding systems were used to describe diseases within epidemiology. Schemes of this type are ICD-9 and ICD-10. They provide a code made up of letters and numbers for just about every disease on the planet. They form a kind of Esperanto for epidemiologists.

Different communities have developed their own coding schema for the different types of information relevant to their needs for recording diagnoses, procedures and medications

Five reasons why coding is essential

Codes provide unambiguous information suitable for computer processing.

Codes allow standard data to be collected across a population.

Codes allow the definition and implementation of standard clinical guidelines and protocols across a group of dental practices in a city, region or even country

Codes allow the collection of standard datasets for performance monitoring and clinical governance.

Coding facilitates comparison between and within practices.

Table 14 Five reasons why coding is essential

Some activities lend themselves to coding and have been long used by dental practices. These are things which are unambiguous and may be mapped onto a single code in such a way as there can be little debate about them. The codes shown in Table 16 were defined for public dentistry in the UK by the NHS Modernisation Agency as a core data set, to be used uniformly across the participating practices

But why should you care as a dentist?

1. If you want to share data, then you have to use the same codes.

2. If you want colleagues in your practice to be able to treat the patient, they will need to be able to interpret your coded data correctly

But the really important reason is:

3. If are paid by an external body such as an insurance company or public health authority on a fee for service basis and you want to be paid for the work that has been done, then your funder must be able to interpret your codes correctly.

For this reason, it is often funders who have the leverage to achieve common standards for coding. They have their own reasons for wanting the information in a form in which it may be analysed:

Five things funders want to do with information

1. Check that your claims are accurate and reasonable

2. Monitor total costs

3. Evaluate high cost areas

4. Check that capacity is sufficient to meet need.

5. Monitor the quality of the activity.

Table 15 Five things funders want to do with information

Topic	Text description	Code
Patient Address	Postcode defines the address to a small number of houses	Postcode
Postcode not supplied	Patient is of no fixed abode.	9085(1)
	Traveller Patient is from a travelling community.	9085(2)
	Visitor to area Patient is visiting from abroad.	9085(3)
	The patient's home postcode is unknown.	9085(4)

New Patient	Patient is new to the practice, ie not seen in the previous 2 years	9082
Method of Entry into the Practice	NHS Direct Patient received practice details from NHS Direct.	9095 (1)
	GMP Patient received practice details from their GP.	9095 (2)
	Self-Referring using Patient received practice details and NHS information or information from PALS or local PCT.	9095 (3)
	Self-Referral from Patient received personal recommendation existing user of practice from friend or family	9095 (4)
	CDS Patient received practice details from Community Dental Service.	9095 (5)
	Other eg patient found practice details in Yellow Pages.	9095 (6)
Patient type	Emergency The clinical opinion is that the patient requires treatment within 24hrs and the patient is not currently within a course of treatment.	9081(3)
	Urgent – unplanned Used for a patient who is undergoing a course of treatment but where, in the opinion of the dentist, treatment not part of the original treatment plan has to be carried out within 24hrs.	9081(4)
	Non-Urgent unplanned Used for a patient who is undergoing a course of treatment but where, in the opinion of the dentist, treatment not part of the original treatment plan has to be carried out soon but not necessarily within 24hrs.	9081(5)
	Routine Normal appointment (eg recall).	9081(6)
	Drop in Patient asking for non-urgent, unplanned treatment or advice. Includes speculative unregistered patients.	9081(7)
Type of Referrals out of Practice	Patient referred to CDS.	9120(1)
	GDS Patient referred to GDS practice.	9120(2)
	PDS Patient referred to other PDS practice.	9120(3)
	Orthodontic Practitioner Patient referred to orthodontic practitioner.	9120(4)
	Patient referred to oral and max-fax specialist.	9120(5)

	Orthodontic Specialist Patient referred to orthodontic specialist.	9120 (6)
	Paediatrics Patient referred to paediatric specialist.	9120(7)
	Periodontal Patient referred to periodontal specialist.	9120(8)
Who provided care for the patient?	Number of contacts with a dentist during a course of treatment	9076(0-99)
	Number of contacts with a dental specialist during a course of treatment: this includes dentists with a specialist interest (endodontic, orthodontic, oral surgery, domiciliary) & not necessarily on the Specialist Register.	9123(0-99)
	Number of contacts with oral health educator during a course of treatment	9079(0-99)
	Number of contacts with a nurse during a course of treatment	9122 (0-99)
	Number of contacts with a professional complimentary to dentistry during a course of treatment	9119 (1-99)
Type of service provided over course of treatment	Restorative All dental treatments excluding preventative. Includes dentures and extractions.	9121(1)
	Preventative A clinical intervention with the aim of preventing future dental problems or where an examination of the patient's mouth takes place but no procedure is undertaken. Examples include check ups, scale and polishes, and procedures such as sealants and varnishes.	9121(2)
	Informative Where healthcare professional has given a patient non-invasive clinical advice with the aim of preventing future dental problems, including smoking cessation sessions.	9121(3)

Table 16 Minimum data set from the English NHS modernisation agency

Web link

There is more information about this available from a link at the website accompanying the book.

The reduction of a traditional text-based record to a structured record can be quite striking. Consider the following episode of care as it is recorded in a traditional hand written record.

3rd February 2005	New patient. Referred by GP. Made appointment for initial assessment visit
24th February 2005	First appointment. Check up. Scale and polish. Referred patient to oral hygienist
22nd April 2005	Patient visited oral hygienist. Discussed smoking cessation. Referred to nurse in charge of programme
12th May 2005	First appointment with smoking cessation nurse
31st May 2005	Second appointment with smoking cessation nurse
14th June 2005	Third appointment with smoking cessation nurse
7th July 2005	6 monthly check up. Scale and polish

is reduced to

Date entered	Codes			
3rd February 2005	9085(4)	9095 (2)		
24th February 2005	9081 (6)			
22nd April 2005	9079(1)			
14th June 2005	9122 (3)			
7th July 2005	9081 (6)	9076(2)	9121(2)	9121(3)

Figure 2 Reducing a handwritten record to a structured record

Now computers love this sort of thing. Even some people who work with computers love this sort of thing, but as an aide-memoire to a practising dentist, it's not great! It contains basic activity information only and does not provide information on the nature of treatment, medications prescribed and other essential information. However, all of this must be coded to consistent and agreed standards if it is to be usefully shared and extracted later. (sorry for the pun!)

☑ Exercise 6

Here's a written record for you to codify. Translate the following record into a coded record using the codes in the Modernisation Agency minimum dataset

---

3rd January 2005	New patient. Self referred after personal recommendation by existing patient. Post code PR1 2HE. Made appointment for initial assessment visit
24th January 2005	First appointment. Check up. Scale and polish. Referred patient to orthodontist
22nd February 2005	Patient visited orthodontist. Discussed programme of treatment
12th March 2005	First appointment with orthodontist
31st March 2005	Second appointment with orthodontist
14th April 2005	Third appointment with orthodontist
7th June 2005	6 monthly check up. Scale and polish

Date entered	Codes			

So for the future, we need a single standard set of agreed codes that can cover diagnoses, signs, symptoms and complaints. This will provide the means not only for

---

diagnostic coding, but when collected compiled and analysed, reliable diagnostic treatment outcomes data can be compiled as well as billing and activity data.

Across the world, health care systems are adopting SNOMED CT as a global coding schema for all aspects of health care. So far it has been adopted in principle by Australia, Canada, Denmark, Lithuania, New Zealand, United Kingdom and the United States although grass roots adoption is very slow.

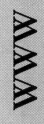

Web link

There is more information about SNOMED CT available from a link at the website accompanying the book.

The American Dental Association has developed SNODENT as a subset of SNOMED CT to be a systematised nomenclature of dentistry containing dental diagnoses, signs, symptoms, and complaints. SNOMED CT includes all the dental terms developed in the UK as part of the Read Code system. It is incompletely integrated into SNOMED CT. Independent scrutiny by Goldberg et al (2005)[6] indicates that currently SNODENT and SNOMED CT are about 85% compatible. In spite of this, they suggest that SNODENT should become the standard dental terminology in the future.

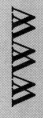

Web link

The presentation slides are available from a link at the website accompanying the book.

For SNODENT to achieve its potential, a number of things need to happen. There is an increasing recognition that oral health can be used as a useful indicator for more general health and as an early warning mechanism for some serious health problems eg cancers.

---

[6] *Louis J. Goldberg, Werner Ceusters, John Eisner, Barry Smith, The Significance of SNODENT, presented at MIE2005, Geneva, Switzerland*

For this reason health care funders are likely to increasingly use incentives to persuade dentists to record their data in a form that can be shared across the health care system and sorted, searched and analysed using standard protocols.

Five things that need to happen to SNODENT

1. It needs to be harmonised with SNOMED CT and recognised as the dental subsection of the larger schema

2. It needs to be adopted as a mandated standard by all agencies responsible for remuneration

3. It needs to be incorporated into computer systems for electronic dental records.

4. It needs to be adopted by dentists, which will happen if the previous two steps happen

5. It needs to be accepted by the wider health care community, and by the international partners involved with SNOMED CT.

Table 17 Five things that need to happen to SNODENT

To see how this might work in practice, supposing you wished to find all the adult female patients who had complained of tooth sensitivity.

The SNODENT code corresponding to tooth sensitivity is D5-10578, so the computer enquiry would become something like:

IF (age >18) AND (sex = female) AND (D5-10578 = found) THEN

WRITELN (Forename, Surname, PatientID)

In practice, of course, it would be more complicated, something like the following which would break the results down by age:

```
'*QRY_WDATE,20071007,07/10/2007'
'*QRY_SDATE,20071007,07/10/2007'
'*QRY_ORDER,001'
'*QRY_TITLE,AGESEX,age–sex breakdown for practice'
'*ENQ_RSPID,UNKNOWN,Unknown respondent'
'*QRY_MEDIA,D,Disk'
'*QRY_AGREE,UNKNOWN,Unknown agreement'
'*QRY_SETID,READ5AGE,Tooth sensitivity amongst adult female patients '
```

```
'*ENQ_IDENT,Anytown Practice,Senior Partner'

'DEFINE AGE AS @YEARS("11/05/2007",DATE_OF_BIRTH)'

ANALYSE

D5-10578

'GROUPED_BY AGE ("0"-"4";"5"-"9";"10"-"14";"15"-"19";"20"-"24";"25"-
"29";"30"-"34"\'

';"35"-"39";"40"-"44";"45"-"49";"50"-"54";"55"-"59";"60"-"64";"65"-"69";"70"\'

'-"74";"75"-"79";"80"-"84";"85"-"89";"90"-"94";"95"-"99";"100"-"104";"105"\'

'-"109")'

FROM PATIENTS
```

Table 18 Sample query to produce a query group by age

Fortunately most of this complex should be hidden from you by your computer system, which should allow you to construct your query from a series of drop down lists.

Why bother?

The American Dental Association has backed the adoption of SNODENT. They argue that SNODENT code usage could allow for:

- National collection of data via clearing houses to analyze treatment outcomes
- Recording a complete oral risk assessment of the patient
- Use of a single code for synonymous descriptive terms, improved claim processing to help reduce or eliminate narrative descriptions or other claim attachments
- In-office monitoring of production and treatment

The problem with pictures

Images are an integral part of dentistry. Images have a fundamental problem for computers. Computers store images as a series of points or "picture elements", often abbreviated to pixels. Each point only has meaning because its context, its relationships with the points around it. When a human being views the image they see a pattern, which is made up of the relationships between the points, not the points themselves. In spite of the limitations of the computer representations of images

On the other hand, digital imaging systems are expensive to install, staff will need re-training, and as with other systems unless the images are stored in a standard way, the images will be reduced to a meaningless stream of numbers when they leave their own systems.

Early digital imaging systems for dentistry tended to store their images in proprietary formats, equivalent to storing a document as a Microsoft Word document. Unless the person receiving the image has the same proprietary application, they can't read the document.

Fortunately, in recent years, a standard has been widely adopted not just for dental images but for other medical images, allowing dentists to share and transmit images even if their imaging systems have come from different manufacturers. This standard is known as DICOM (Digital Imaging and Communications in Medicine). DICOM was born out of the work of a joint committee of The American College of Radiology (ACR) and the National Electrical Manufacturers Association (NEMA), formed in 1983 to develop a standard to:

- Promote communication of digital image information, regardless of device manufacturer

- Facilitate the development and expansion of picture archiving and communication systems (PACS) that can also interface with other systems of hospital information

- Allow the creation of diagnostic information data bases that can be interrogated by a wide variety of devices distributed geographically.

Frankly, DICOM has the same relationship to most dentists as car maintenance does to my driving. I know it's really important, but I don't need to know the details. I employ someone else to do that, and probably pay them handsomely to do it.

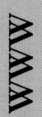

Web link

However, for those of you who can't resist peeking under the bonnet, or just have a bad case of insomnia, full details of the DICOM standard are available from a link at the website accompanying the book.

Advantages of digital X-rays

- Digital systems can improve practice efficiency as they save time in many phases of the dental team's work.

- Digital imaging eliminates waiting times of film processing.

- Digital images can electronically be sent to insurance companies and social security for faster reimbursement.

- Digital practice can be economical in the longer term as costs related to X-ray consumables and the maintenance can be eliminated

- Routine activities are reduced since digital practice requires less maintenance and manual work such as archiving of the patient records, film processor maintenance and handling of film and film cassettes.

- Consistent quality can easily be maintained, since digital X-ray images are not subject to variations and errors typical to film based imaging.

- The user can easily make copies of the images without decreasing the diagnostic quality and the original images are always available.

- Digital X-ray systems offer personnel and patient health and safety advantages: it significantly reduces the patient radiation dose, the practice no longer needs chemical X-ray film processing, which occupies space, produces odors and chemical waste, which is difficult to dispose.

- Digital technology can have a positive effect on the practice image. Digital technology is perceived as 'hitech' and practices using digital equipment may be perceived as quality oriented, modern and conscientious.

Table 19 Advantages of digital X-rays

☑ Exercise 7

Think about your own practice. What are the barriers and motivators to adopting a standard coding scheme like SNODENT, and are they major or minor?

Barriers	Major or minor?	Motivators	Major or minor?

Think Box

Before we leave this chapter think about the following question:

What information is held by other health care professionals that would be useful to you?

What information that would be useful to other health care professionals is held by you?

Would you be prepared to share it, and if so, under what conditions?

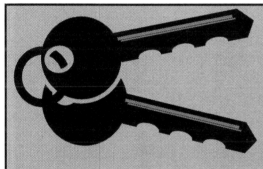

Key points from this chapter

Codes are probably the second most important thing to get right about your information solution for your dental practice

Computers can process information quickly, but only if it is clear and unambiguous

Coding systems meet a need to describe the world of healthcare in concise and unambiguous ways, that is essential for the effective use of computers

Much of the complexity of coding and terminology can be hidden inside the computer system once defined

It is essential for the sharing of information to define and adhere to coding standards

Chapter 6 Patient privacy

Within the UK public health care system, a system of governance has developed in respect of handling information

Information Governance is guided by five basic principles on the protection and use of patient information:

Five basic principles on the protection and use of patient information

- Don't use patient information unless absolutely necessary.

- Use the minimum necessary.

- Access on a strict need-to-know basis.

- Be aware of responsibilities.

- Understand and comply with the law.

Table 20 Five basic principles on the protection and use of patient information

These principles are derived from legislative and professional responsibilities, and apply across public and private dental care and across different countries. We shall consider first the UK context, but then consider the North American context

It is not specifically an IT issue. However, the increased adoption of IT and clinical staff's occasional unfamiliarity with it can raise particular governance issues. It makes it easier to store and distribute information for better and for worse.

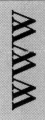

Web link

There is a link provided to the government agencies responsible for privacy and data protection from the website accompanying the book

The first UK Data Protection Act was established in 1984 to deal with protection of data held on computers. In 1998, this was replaced by a much more comprehensive Act which brought us into line with Europe.

The major differences in the 1998 Act, which actually became law in 2000, are as follows:

Five new things in the 1998 UK Data Protection Act

- the Act now covers certain types of manual records (including all health records) as well as electronic records. There are transitional arrangements concerning manual records between now and 2007;

- the definition of 'processing' is wider than that in the 1984 Act, and includes the concepts of obtaining, storing and disclosing data. Most actions involving data, including storage, will be included within this definition;

- although both the 1984 and 1998 Act include eight Data Protection Principles, the nature of the principles differs between the two Acts;

- the Access to Health Records Act 1990 permitted access to manual health records made after the Act came into force (1 November 1991). The Data Protection Act 1998 permits access to all manual health records whenever made, subject to specified exceptions;

- changes to the requirements for notification of processing to the Data Protection Commissioner (formerly the Data Protection Registrar).

Guidance on the 1998 Act, Department of Health

Table 21 Five new things in the 1998 UK Data Protection Act

UK law now states that anyone processing personal data must comply with the eight enforceable principles of good practice:.

Personal data covers both facts and opinions about the individual. It also includes information regarding the intentions of the data controller towards the individual, although in some limited circumstances exemptions will apply. With processing, the definition is far wider than before.

All processing of data to which the Act applies must comply with the eight principles. The first principle is particularly important as it emphasises that processing must be fair and lawful in the context of the common law and other UK legislation.

The Eight Data Protection Principles

Data must be:

- fairly and lawfully processed;

- processed for limited purposes;

- adequate, relevant and not excessive;

- accurate;

- not kept longer than necessary;

- processed in accordance with the data subject's rights;

- secure;

- not transferred to countries without adequate protection.

Source:, UK Information Commissioner

Table 22 The Eight Data Protection Principles

Generally it will be complied with if all the following conditions are met:

- the common law of confidentiality and any other applicable statutory restrictions on the use of information are complied with;

- the data subject was not misled or deceived into giving the data;

- the data subject is given basic information about who will process the data and or what purpose;

- in the case of health data, one of the conditions in both Schedule 2, which deals with any personal data, and Schedule 3 to the Act, which deals with sensitive personal data is satisfied.

Think Box

Before we leave this section think about the following question:

Are you sure you are operating within the law?

According to the UK General Dental Council, one of the six key ethical principles dentists should follow is:

Protecting patients' confidential information

This principle sets out the need to treat information about patients as confidential, using it only for the purposes for which it was given. Dental professionals should also take steps to prevent accidental disclosure or unauthorised access to confidential information by keeping information secure at all times.

In some limited circumstances disclosure of confidential patient information without consent may be justified in the public interest (for example to assist in the prevention or detection of a serious crime) or may be required by law or by Court order. Dental professionals should seek appropriate advice before disclosing information on this basis.

Standards for dental professionals, ethical guidance, UK General Dental Council

Table 23 Protecting patients' confidential information

The first issue arising from this principle is: what constitutes confidential information?

Within the UK NHS, it is defined thus:

A duty of confidence arises when one person discloses information to another (eg patient to clinician) in circumstances where it is reasonable to expect that the information will be held in confidence. It -

1. is a legal obligation that is derived from case law;

2. is a requirement established within professional codes of conduct; and

3. must be included within NHS employment contracts as a specific requirement linked to disciplinary procedures.

Confidentiality: NHS Code of Practice, HMSO, London, 2003

Is that helpful? I thought not!

The official guidance makes a distinction between patient identifiable data and non-identifiable data. This creates its own set of difficulties.

Anonymised data may still be identifiable from other factors. For example, it would be difficult to identify a patient from a diagnosis of asthma, as this is very common.

As we refine the diagnosis, and combine it with other factors such as age gender and ethnicity, we may quickly provide a unique profile of a patient, who could be identified.

In practice, the duty of care on a clinician to protect the data is not removed by anonymising it. Some of the anonymised data used routinely for disease surveillance in public health, including for example sexually transmitted disease data, is amongst the most sensitive.

Alternatively, if we diagnose a rare condition, that may be unique within a practice or locality

The Department of Health guidance on confidentiality states that:

The UK Department of Health guidance on confidentiality

It is extremely important that patients are made aware of information disclosures that must take place in order to provide them with high quality care. In particular, clinical governance and clinical audits, which are wholly proper components of healthcare provision, might not be obvious to patients and should be drawn to their attention. Similarly, whilst patients may understand that information needs to be shared between members of care teams and between different organisations involved in healthcare provision, this may not be the case and the efforts made to inform them should reflect the breadth of the required disclosure. This is particularly important where disclosure extends to non-NHS bodies.

Confidentiality: NHS Code of Practice, HMSO, London, 2003

Table 24 The UK Department of Health guidance on confidentiality

The grey area in all these cases comes where patients refuse to give consent for disclosure of information. Clinicians may be faced with a choice between doing the best for their patient and their obligations to the broader healthcare system. The official advice seems to me to plausible but fails to deal with the complexities faced by clinicians in practice:

Advice from the NHS Code of Practice, HMSO, London, 2003

Patients generally have the right to object to the use and disclosure of confidential information that identifies them, and need to be made aware of this right. Sometimes, if patients choose to prohibit information being disclosed to other health professionals involved in providing care, it might mean that the care that can be provided is limited and, in extremely rare circumstances, that it is not possible to offer certain treatment options. Patients must be informed if their decisions about disclosure have implications for the provision of care or treatment. Clinicians cannot usually treat patients safely, nor provide continuity of care, without having relevant information about a patient's condition and medical history.

Confidentiality: NHS Code of Practice, HMSO, London, 2003

Table 25 Advice from the NHS Code of Practice, HMSO, London, 2003

For example, clinicians find themselves all the time with inadequate information, balancing that against the good of the patient, eg in drop in centres, NHS Direct and when called out at night

Ultimately, the law does state that there are situations where consent cannot be obtained for the use or disclosure of patient identifiable information, yet the public good of this use outweighs issues of privacy. Section 60 of the Health and Social Care Act 2001 currently provides an interim power to ensure that patient identifiable information, needed to support a range of important work such as clinical audit, record validation and research, can be used without the consent of patients.

When a patient discloses private information to their dentist, or another individual clinician, they do not necessarily expect that information to be available to another member of their healthcare team.

They may go further and explicitly state that they wish it remain confidential to that individual clinician. In the modern healthcare system, however, care is often a team activity and may require information sharing amongst the team.

The official advice states:

UK NHS advice on team confidentiality

Patients generally have the right to object to the use and disclosure of confidential information that identifies them, and the need to be made aware of this right. Sometimes if patients choose to prohibit information being disclosed to other health professionals involved in providing care, it might mean that the care that can be offered can be limited and in extremely rare circumstances that it is not possible to offer certain treatment options. Patients must be informed if their decisions about disclosure have implications for the provision of care or treatment.

Confidentiality: NHS Code of Practice, HMSO, London, 2003

Table 26 UK NHS advice on team confidentiality

Most patients would be happy to share more personal information with their own dentist than with another clinician. Equally, they would be happier to share it with a clinician who is directly involved in their treatment than one who is not, or a manager who is using the information for a purpose that has a less direct impact upon the care of that patient. In other systems, eg Australia, where there is a much weaker link between patients and a specific clinician, the emphasis upon patient privacy is stronger.

An Australian Experience

On a recent visit, I interviewed a GP about his patients, many of whom had serious conditions including HIV/AIDS. He said:

'My patients would come to me for treatment relating to their AIDS or hepatitis. They would visit another GP closer to home for their routine medication, and that physician may not know of their condition.'

(Australian GP)

This raised serious issues for me around the balance between confidentiality and the risk to the patients' health. Upon return to the UK, I queried this with a UK GP, and asked him if the position was similar here. He replied that:

'If a patient is diagnosed with a condition such as AIDS by an outside agency, for example an STD clinic, that diagnosis would not necessarily be reported to their GP.'

(UK GP)

Whilst this reflects a vital sensitivity to the need for confidentiality around diseases which may carry a significant stigma in society, it undermines the principle that UK GPs have overall responsibility for the care of their patients, and that this principle is not necessarily carried over to other conditions that may carry equal stigma, eg mental health problems.

Extract from Gillies, AC (2003) What is a good health care system, Radcliffe Publishing

Table 27 An Australian experience

There is a clear trade-off between disclosure of information to professional colleagues on a 'Need-to-know' basis and the desire for patient privacy. However, there is a clear principle that patients' consent must be sought for disclosure, and that that consent must be properly informed.

Increasingly, patient care is a multi-agency activity, involving several health agencies, social care agencies and, increasingly, voluntary agencies. Dentists are increasingly encouraged to link up care and information with other health care professionals. There is a tension between providing the best possible information, especially in a multi-agency situation to facilitate the best possible care and the need to respect confidentiality.

As defined in the UK Data Protection Act 1998, medical (including dental) purposes include but are wider than healthcare purposes. They include preventative activity, research, financial audit and management of healthcare services. The Health and Social Care Act 2001 explicitly broadened the definition to include social care.

More recent policy has increasingly treated social care as part of healthcare. However, this does not cover other agencies eg voluntary agencies or the police. Whilst the police have no general right of access to health records, there are a number of statutes which require disclosure to them and some that permit disclosure. These have the effect of making disclosure a legitimate function in the circumstances they cover. In the absence of a requirement to disclose there must be either explicit patient consent or a robust public interest justification. What is or isn't in the public interest is ultimately decided by the courts. Where disclosure is justified it should be limited to the minimum necessary to meet the need and patients should be informed of the disclosure unless it would defeat the purpose of the investigation, allow a potential criminal to escape or put staff or others at risk.

UK Department of Health guidance on joint working

The guidance highlights the following principles:

- information to be shared must be purposeful and justified;

- information should be specifically geared to the task it is intended to serve;

- the information should be sufficient and sharing should exclude unnecessary material;

- information should normally only be shared with the informed consent of the subject;

- information should be shared as part of appropriately planned and managed procedures;

- information should only be shared within agreed 'information communities';

- personal identifiers should be removed wherever possible;

- agencies should take responsibility for ensuring proper procedures for compliance;

- standards must be established to ensure that technologies used in information sharing are fully fit for the purpose.

Draft guidance and regulations on the section 31 partnership arrangements, 1999

Table 28 UK Department of Health guidance on joint working

Most NHS organisations will have procedures to deal with such situations, and dentists working in this sector should refer to these to protect themselves and their patients.

Since the underlying principles are determined by universal ethical principles, the situation in North America is not dissimilar.

In the US, the first-ever federal privacy standards to protect patients' records and other health information provided to health plans, doctors, dentists, hospitals and other health care providers were implemented on April 14, 2003. The standards were developed by the Department of Health and Human Services (HHS). They provide patients with access to their medical records and more control over how their personal health information is used and disclosed. They represent a uniform, federal minimum level of privacy protection for consumers throughout the country.

State laws providing additional protections to consumers are not affected by these rules.

The HHS were required by Congress to issue patient privacy protections as part of the Health Insurance Portability and Accountability Act of 1996 (HIPAA). HIPAA included provisions designed to encourage electronic transactions and also required new safeguards to protect the security and confidentiality of health information.

Privacy rules for US Dentists

- Access To Dental Records. Patients generally should be able to see and obtain copies of their dental records and request corrections if they identify errors and mistakes. Health plans, doctors, hospitals, clinics, nursing homes and other covered entities generally should provide access these records within 30 days and may charge patients for the cost of copying and sending the records.

- Notice of Privacy Practices. Covered health plans, doctors and other health care providers must provide a notice to their patients how they may use personal dental information and their rights under the new privacy regulation.. Patients generally will be asked to sign, initial or otherwise acknowledge that they received this notice.. Patients may also ask covered entities to restrict the use or disclosure of their information beyond the practices included in the notice, but the covered entities would not have to agree to the changes.

- Limits on Use of Personal Dental Information. The privacy rule sets limits on how health plans and covered providers may use individually identifiable health information. To promote the best quality care for patients, the rule does not restrict the ability of doctors, nurses and other providers to share information needed to treat their patients. In other situations, though, personal health information generally may not be used for purposes not related to health care, and covered entities may use or share only the minimum amount of protected information needed for a particular purpose. In addition, patients would have to sign a specific authorization before a covered entity could release their dental information to a life insurer, a bank, a marketing firm or another outside business for purposes not related to their health care.

- Prohibition on Marketing. The final privacy rule sets restrictions and limits on the use of patient information for marketing purposes. Pharmacies, health plans and other covered entities must first obtain an individual's specific authorization before disclosing their patient information for marketing. At the same time, the rule permits doctors and other covered entities to communicate freely with patients about treatment options and other health-related information, including disease-management programs.

- Stronger State Laws. The federal privacy standards do not affect state laws that provide additional privacy protections for patients. The confidentiality protections are cumulative; the privacy rule will set a national "floor" of privacy standards that protect all Americans, and any state law providing additional protections would continue to apply. When a state law requires a certain disclosure - such as reporting an infectious disease outbreak to the public health authorities - the federal privacy regulations would not over-rule the state law.

- Confidential communications. Under the privacy rule, patients can request that their dentists, health plans and other covered entities take reasonable steps to ensure that their communications with the patient are confidential. For example, a patient could ask a dentist to call his or her office rather than home, and the doctor's office should comply with that request if it can be reasonably accommodated.

- Complaints. Consumers may file a formal complaint regarding the privacy practices of a covered health plan or provider. Such complaints can be made directly to the covered provider or health plan or to HHS' Office for Civil Rights (OCR), which is charged with investigating complaints and enforcing the privacy regulation. Information about filing complaints should be included in each covered entity's notice of privacy practices.

Table 29 US 2003 Privacy rules as defined within the HIPAA regulations

The final regulations cover health plans, health care clearinghouses, and those health care providers who conduct certain financial and administrative transactions (eg enrolment, billing and eligibility verification) electronically.The 2003 privacy regulations ensure a national floor of privacy protections for patients by limiting the ways that health plans, pharmacies, hospitals and other covered entities can use patients' personal dental information. The regulations protect dental records and other individually identifiable health information, whether it is on paper, in computers or communicated orally.

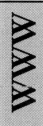

Web link

There is a link provided to the privacy section of HHS web site from the website accompanying the book.

The privacy rule requires health plans, dentists, pharmacies, doctors and other covered entities to establish policies and procedures to protect the confidentiality of protected health information about their patients. These requirements are flexible and scalable to allow different covered entities to implement them as appropriate for their businesses or practices. Covered entities must provide all the protections for patients cited above, such as providing a notice of their privacy practices and limiting the use and disclosure of information as required under the rule. In addition, covered entities must take some additional steps to protect patient privacy:

- Written Privacy Procedures. The rule requires covered entities to have written privacy procedures, including a description of staff that has access to protected information, how it will be used and when it may be disclosed. Covered entities generally must take steps to ensure that any business associates who have access to protected information agree to the same limitations on the use and disclosure of that information.

- Employee Training and Privacy Officer. Covered entities must train their employees in their privacy procedures and must designate an individual to be responsible for ensuring the procedures are followed. If covered entities learn an employee failed to follow these procedures, they must take appropriate disciplinary action.

- Public Responsibilities. In limited circumstances, the final rule permits -- but does not require --covered entities to continue certain existing disclosures of health information for specific public responsibilities. These permitted disclosures include: emergency circumstances; identification of the body of a deceased person, or the cause of death; public health needs; research that involves limited data or has been independently approved by an Institutional Review Board or privacy board; oversight of the health care system; judicial and administrative proceedings; limited law enforcement activities; and activities related to national defense and security. The privacy rule generally establishes safeguards and limits on these disclosures. Where no other law requires disclosures in these situations, covered entities may continue to use their professional judgment to decide whether to make such disclosures based on their own policies and ethical principles.

- Equivalent Requirements For Government. The provisions of the final rule generally apply equally to private sector and public sector covered entities. For example, private hospitals and government-run hospitals covered by the rule have to comply with the full range of requirements.

The following is a sample statement for a University Dental School: most dental practices will have less functions to cover than this.

US Sample privacy statement from a University dental school

NOTICE OF PRIVACY PRACTICES

Effective Date _____

UNIVERSITY OF _____ SCHOOL OF DENTAL MEDICINE

THIS NOTICE DESCRIBES HOW DENTAL INFORMATION ABOUT YOU MAY BE USED AND DISCLOSED AND HOW YOU CAN GET ACCESS TO THIS INFORMATION. PLEASE REVIEW IT CAREFULLY.

YOU WILL BE ASKED TO ACKNOWLEDGE THAT YOU HAVE RECEIVED OUR NOTICE OF PRIVACY PRACTICES.

We understand that information about you and your health is very personal and therefore, we will strive to protect your privacy as required by law. We will only use and disclose your personal health information as allowed by applicable law.

We are committed to excellence in the provision of state-of-the-art health care services through the practice of patient care, education, and research. Therefore, as described below, your health information will be used to provide you care and may be used to educate health care professionals and for research. We train our staff and workforce to be sensitive about privacy and to respect the confidentiality of your personal health information.

We are required by law to maintain the privacy of our patients' personal health information and to provide patients with notice of our legal duties and privacy practices with respect to your personal health information. We are required to abide by the terms of this Notice of Privacy Practices so long as it remains in effect. We reserve the right to change the terms of this Notice of Privacy Practices as necessary and to make the new Notice of Privacy Practices effective for all personal health information maintained by us. You may receive a copy of any revised notice at any SDM registration area or on the Internet at http://www.dental.____.edu/npp/ or a copy may be obtained by mailing a request to:

Chief Privacy Officer; School of Dental Medicine; University of _____;

The terms of this Notice of Privacy Practices apply to:

- All departments and units of the School of Dental Medicine (SDM), including the Dental Care Network (DCN).

- All employees, staff and other SDM personnel.

- Any healthcare professional we authorize to enter information into your dental chart.

- Any member of a volunteer group we allow to help you while you are in the SDM.

This Notice of Privacy Practices does not apply to care you receive in dentists' private offices.

USES AND DISCLOSURES OF YOUR PERSONAL HEALTH INFORMATION

The following categories detail the various ways in which we may use or disclose your personal health information. For each category of uses or disclosures we will give you illustrative examples. It should be noted that while not every use or disclosure will be listed, each of the ways we are permitted to use or disclose information will fall into one of the following categories.

Your Authorization. Except as outlined below, we will not use or disclose your personal health information for any purpose unless you have signed a form authorizing the use or disclosure. This form will describe what information will be disclosed, to whom, for what purpose, and when. You have the right to revoke that authorization in writing, except to the extent we have already relied upon it.

For Treatment. We may use dental information about you to provide you with dental treatment or services. We may disclose dental information about you to dentists, technicians, dental students, or other SDM personnel who are involved in taking care of you at the SDM. For example, a dentist treating you may need to know if you have diabetes because diabetes may slow the healing process. Different departments of the SDM also may share dental information about you in order to coordinate the care you need, such as prescriptions, lab work and x-rays. We also may disclose dental information about you to people outside the SDM who may be involved in your dental care after you leave the SDM, such as family members or others we use to provide services that are part of your care.

For Payment. We may use and disclose dental information about you so that the treatment and services you receive at the SDM may be billed to and payment may be collected from you, an insurance company or a third party. For example, we may need to give your dental plan information about treatment you received at the SDM so your health plan will pay us or reimburse you for the treatment. We may also tell your dental plan about a treatment you are going to receive to obtain prior approval or to determine whether your plan will cover the treatment.

For Healthcare Operations. We may use and disclose dental information about you for SDM operations. These uses and disclosures are necessary to run the SDM and make sure that all of our patients receive quality care. For example, we may use dental information to review our treatment and services and to evaluate the performance of our staff in caring for you. We may also combine dental information about many SDM patients to decide what additional services the SDM should offer, what services are not needed, and whether certain new treatments are effective. We may also disclose information to dentists, technicians, dental students, and other SDM personnel for review and learning purposes. We may also combine the dental information we have with information from other clinics to compare how we are doing and see where we can make improvements in the care and services we offer. We will remove information that identifies you from this set of dental information so others may use it to study healthcare and healthcare delivery without learning who the specific patients are.

Appointment Reminders. We may use and disclose dental information to contact you as a reminder that you have an appointment for treatment or dental care at the SDM. The reminder may be by mail or as a telephone message.

Treatment Alternatives. We may use and disclose dental information to tell you about or recommend possible treatment options or alternatives that may be of interest to you.

Health-Related Benefits and Services. We may use and disclose dental information to tell you about health-related benefits or services that may be of interest to you.

Fundraising Activities. We may use dental information about you to contact you in an effort to raise money for the SDM and its operations. We may disclose dental information to a foundation related to the SDM so that the foundation may contact you in raising money for the SDM. We only would release contact information, such as your name, address and phone number and the dates you received treatment or services at the SDM. If you do not want the SDM to contact you for fundraising efforts, you must notify the Patient Advocate in writing who may be contacted at 000-000-0000 or through email at pat_adv@pobox.u_____.edu..

Individuals Involved in Your Care or Payment for Your Care. We will only disclose information to a patient's guardian, representative with power of attorney, and to people the patient invites to physically accompany him or her. Information will be disclosed to this patient representative in the presence of the patient. In certain emergency situations it may not be possible to have the patient present, in which case the SDM may, in the exercise of professional judgment, determine whether the disclosure is in the best interests of the patient, and if so, disclose only information directly relevant to the person's involvement with the patient's health care or related payment.

Research. We may use and disclose your personal health information as permitted or required by law, for research, subject to your explicit authorization, and/or oversight by the University of Pennsylvania Institutional Review Boards, committees charged with protecting the privacy rights and safety of human subject research, or a similar committee. In all cases where your specific authorization has not been obtained, your privacy will be protected by confidentiality requirements evaluated by such committee. This is necessary to investigate cutting-edge health care through improved treatments, medications and outcomes research. For example, you may be approached by your dentist to ask if you would be interested in participating in a clinical trial of a new drug for your condition. Or, your health information may be used with the approval of the committee charged with protecting the rights of research subjects, described above, to conduct outcomes research to see if a particular procedure is effective.

Business Associates. Certain aspects and components of our services are performed through contracts with outside persons or organizations, such as auditing, accreditation, legal services, etc. At times it may be necessary for us to provide certain of your personal health information to one or more of these outside persons or organizations who assist us with our payment/billing activities and health care operations. In such cases, we require these business associates to appropriately safeguard the privacy of your information.

Other Uses and Disclosures. We are permitted or required by law to make certain other uses and disclosures of your personal health information without your consent or authorization. Subject to conditions specified by law:

- We may release your personal health information for any purpose required by law;

- We may release your personal health information for public health activities, such as required reporting of disease, injury, and birth and death, and for required public health investigations;

- We may release your personal health information to certain governmental agencies if we suspect child abuse or neglect; we may also release your personal health information to certain governmental agencies if we believe you to be a victim of abuse, neglect, or domestic violence;

- We may release your personal health information to entities regulated by the Food and Drug Administration if necessary to report adverse, product defects, or to participate in product recalls;

- We may release your personal health information to your employer when we have provided health care to you at the request of your employer for purposes related to occupational health and safety; in most cases you will receive notice that information is disclosed to your employer;

- We may release your personal health information if required by law to a government oversight agency conducting audits, investigations, inspections and related oversight functions;

- We may use or disclose your personal health information in emergency circumstances, such as to prevent a serious and imminent threat to a person or the public;

- We may release your personal health information if required to do so by a court or administrative order, subpoena or discovery request; in most cases you will have notice of such release;

- We may release your personal health information to law enforcement officials to identify or locate suspects, fugitives or witnesses, or victims of crime, or for other allowable law enforcement purposes;

- We may release your personal health information to coroners, medical examiners, and/or funeral directors;

- We may release your personal health information if necessary to arrange an organ or tissue donation from you or a transplant for you;

- We may release your personal health information if you are a member of the military for activities set out by certain military command authorities as required by armed forces services; we may also release your personal health information if necessary for national security, intelligence, or protective services activities; and

- We may release your personal health information if necessary for purposes related to your workers' compensation benefits.

Confidentiality of Alcohol and Drug Abuse Patient Records, HIV-Related Information, and Mental Health Records. The confidentiality of alcohol and drug abuse patient records, HIV-related information, and mental health records maintained by us is specifically protected by state and/or Federal law and regulations. Generally, we may not disclose such information unless you consent in writing, the disclosure is allowed by a court order, or in limited and regulated other circumstances.

RIGHTS THAT YOU HAVE

Access to Your Personal Health Information. Generally, you have the right to access, inspect, and/or copy personal health information that we maintain about you. Requests for access must be made in writing and be signed by you or your representative. We will charge you for a copy of your medical records in accordance with a schedule of fees established by applicable state law. You may obtain an access request form from the SDM Patient Advocate who may be contacted at 000-000-0000 or through email at pat_adv@pobox.u_____.edu..

Amendments to Your Personal Health Information. You have the right to request that personal health information that we maintain about you be amended or corrected. We are not obligated to make all requested amendments but will give each request careful consideration. All amendment requests, in order to be considered by us, must be in writing, signed by you or your representative, and must state the reasons for the amendment/correction request. If an amendment or correction you request is made by us, we may also notify others who work with us and have copies of the uncorrected record if we believe that such notification is necessary. Please note that even if we accept your request, we may not delete any information already documented in your medical record. You may obtain an amendment request form from the SDM Patient Advocate who may be contacted at 215-573-4742 or through email at pat_adv@pobox.u_____.edu.

Accounting for Disclosures of Your Personal Health Information. You have the right to receive an accounting of certain disclosures made by us of your personal health information after April 14, 2003 except for disclosures made for purposes of treatment, payment, and healthcare operations or for certain other limited exceptions. Requests must be made in writing and signed by you or your representative. Accounting request forms are available from the SDM Patient Advocate who may be contacted at 000-000-

0000 or through email at pat_adv@pobox.u_____.edu.. The first accounting in any 12-month period is free; you will be charged a fee for each subsequent accounting you request within the same 12-month period. We will notify you of the cost involved and you may choose to withdraw or modify your request at that time before any costs are incurred.

Restrictions on Use and Disclosure of Your Personal Health Information. You have the right to request restrictions on certain of our uses and disclosures of your personal health information for treatment, payment, or health care operations. For example, you may request that we do not share your health information with a certain family member. A restriction request form can be obtained from the SDM Patient Advocate who may be contacted at 000-000-0000 or through email at pat_adv@pobox.u_____.edu. We are not required to agree to your restriction request but will attempt to accommodate reasonable requests when appropriate and we retain the right to terminate an agreed-to restriction if we believe such termination is appropriate. In the event we have terminated an agreed upon restriction, we will notify you of such termination.

Confidential Communications. You have the right to request communications regarding your personal health information from us by alternative means or at alternative locations and we will accommodate reasonable requests by you. To request confidential communications, you must fill out the Request to Receive Confidential Communication by Alternative Means or at Alternative Locations Form and submit it to the Patient Advocate who may be contacted at 000-000-0000 or through email at pat_adv@pobox.u_____.edu.

Paper Copy of Notice. As a patient you retain the right to obtain a paper copy of this Notice of Privacy Practices, even if you have requested such copy by e-mail or other electronic means. You may also obtain a copy of this notice via the Internet at http://www.dental.u_____.edu/npp/

ADDITIONAL INFORMATION

Complaints. If you believe your privacy rights have been violated, you may file a complaint with the SDM Patient Advocate who may be contacted at 000-000-0000 or through email at pat_adv@pobox.u_____.edu. You may also file a complaint with the Secretary of the U.S. Department of Health and Human Services in Washington D.C. All complaints must be made in writing and in no way will affect the quality of care you receive from us.

For further information. If you have questions or need further assistance regarding this Notice of Privacy Practices, you may contact the Chief Privacy Officer who may be contacted at 215-000-000-0000 or sdm_cpo@pobox.u_____.edu.

Table 30 Sample privacy policy from a US University Dental School

In Canada , the Canadian Dental association provides the following advice:

Dental Records - Confidentiality, Transfer and Third Party Access

Dental records are collections of sensitive personal patient information compiled to allow dentists and other dental health care providers to provide dental treatment, provide continuity of care and maintain optimal standards of care. Original dental records compiled by a dentist are the legal property of the dentist.

Patients have a legal right to examine and copy their records and to control the use and dissemination of the information contained in their records. Dentists require patients to provide complete, accurate and intimate health details in order to provide safe and effective treatment. Therefore, ownership of original dental records obligate the security and confidentiality of this information contained therein which may be developed only with the permission of the patient except when otherwise required by law.

Patients have the right to control disclosure of their dental records to others. Release of information must be informed; must be specific and for a one time event; must afford the patient an opportunity to review that information requested and being released prior to the transfer and with an opportunity to withdraw prior consent; must not be used for any purpose other than the primary and specific use requested; and must be with the patient's permission, preferably in writing.

Patients are entitled to receive dental care in a confidential setting free of third party intrusion. Release of patient information to third parties must adhere to the basic principles of confidentiality and patient rights outlined above with the intention of enabling patients to review any and all third party benefits to which they may be entitled. Patients may be unaware of the information third parties may have access to under broad based consents to release dental records and the scope of this information may exceed the needs of third party to determine benefits. It becomes the responsibility of the dentist and other dental health care providers to protect the confidentiality and privacy of their patients.

Where a third party (eg government agency, Revenue Canada, dental association or insurance company) has received patient permission to use information from the patient's dental records for financial audits, all patient identity and unrelated information (eg health history, personal information) shall first be removed from the records. No third party can demand access to patient dental records (including financial records) except with specific patient consent in writing, by legal statute or by court order.

Table 31 Dental Records - Confidentiality, Transfer and Third Party Access

In Canada, there are provincial as well as federal privacy rules. A sample security policy designed to meet the needs of Ontario privacy legislation is provided below:

Suggested sample privacy policy for Ontario dentists

Introduction

The *Personal Health Information Protection Act, 2004* (the *Act*) requires all custodians of health information to protect personal health information in their custody or control and to ensure that records are retained, transferred and disposed of in a secure manner .

This policy is designed to help practice staff execute this responsibility

Storage of Personal Health Information

The practice and their staff will take reasonable steps to keep personal health information securely stored at all times

The Information and Privacy Commissioner states that steps to ensure safe storage of personal health information should address physical security, technological security and administrative controls .

Practice staff will safeguard physical security by

- Locking personal information held on paper filing cabinets,

- Not leaving information unattended either on paper on an accessible computer

- Locking offices when unattended

- Not leaving patients alone in rooms with access to personal data

- Ensuring that only authorised personnel have keys , and

- Installing and maintaining appropriate alarm systems .

Practice staff will safeguard technological security by

- using passwords to protect sensitive data. passwords will
  - have a mixture of numbers and letters
  - have at least 8 characters
  - be changed at least every quarter

- not transmitting data by unsecured means, either by unencrypted emails, or by fax without first confirming that the recipient is present at the receiving machine in a secure environment

- not introducing unauthorised data or applications into the system which may introduce a virus or other malware.

- using software to lock their system when they leave their workstations unattended and automatically after 5 minutes of inactivity.

- complying with all practice procedures to protect patient data

- ensuring that any data held on mobile devices such as laptops, PDAs or memory sticks will be subject to the same safeguards as the fixed resources.

The practice will safeguard technological and administrative security by

- Deploying firewalls and virus scanners to protect the systems and data .

- Designating a staff member with overall responsibility for security;

- Providing regular staff training;

- Establishing security protocols and access restrictions for designated groups of users

- Carrying out regular audits of actual practices for compliance with security policies; and

- Including confidentiality agreements into employment contracts

- Install automatic back-up for file recovery to protect records from loss or damage; and

- Keep an audit trail that, at a minimum: ·

  - Records the date and time of each entry for each patient; ·

  - Shows any changes in the record; and

  - Preserves the original content when a record is changed, updated or corrected .

Privacy breaches

The practice will notify individuals whose personal health information has been stolen, lost or accessed by an unauthorized person .

Retention of personal health information

The *Act* requires personal health records be kept for as long as needed to allow an individual to exhaust any legal recourse regarding a request for access .

As a best practice, personal health records should be retained for their minimum retention periods .

The practice will establish retention periods for all categories of personal health data.

The practice will carry out regular audits to ensure compliance with the agreed retention schedule.

Transfer of personal health information

The practice will undertake to transfer records to facilities, other practices and their staff or successors .in accordance with the requirements of PHIPA, in pursuant of continuing care for the patient.

The practice and their staff will securely transfer records, in accordance with governing legislation and regulatory procedures to determine appropriate transfer requirements .

The practice and their staff will make reasonable efforts to notify patients before transferring records to a successor, or if that is not reasonably possible, as soon as possible after the transfer .

Disposal of personal health information

The practice and their staff will securely dispose of personal health records, that are no longer retained so that the personal health information cannot be retrieved .

For hard copy records, secure disposal will mean shredding or burning.

For electronic records, secure disposal will mean either physically destroying the media they are stored on (such as a CD) or magnetically erasing or overwriting the information in such a way that the information cannot be recovered .

The practice and their staff will keep a record of disposal dates and the names of individuals whose records were disposed of .

Should the practice require records to be physically moved, the practice will take all reasonable care to keep the data secure and any disposal will follow normal procedures.

If any practice computers are to be sold, all personal health information will first be erased in such a way that it cannot be recovered .

Consent

The practice will comply with Ontario's health privacy legislation, the *Personal Health Information Protection Act* (*PHIPA*).

PHIPA replaces all previous legislation on consent including Form 14. However, a member of the PRACTICE who obtained express consent using a Form 14 before *PHIPA* came into force on November 1, 2004 or a custodian that receives a Form 14 that was executed prior to November 1, 2004, is entitled to assume that it fulfils the requirements of *PHIPA* unless it is not reasonable to assume so.

Consent for the collection, use or disclosure of personal health information is required under *PHIPA*, practice staff will ensure that consent meets the following requirements.

Consent must:

- Relate to the information;

- Be the consent of the individual (or substitute decision-maker, where authorized);

- Be knowledgeable; and

- Not be obtained through coercion or deception (be voluntary).

The "knowledgeable consent" requirement of *PHIPA* means that individuals must know why the information is being collected,

In emergency and limited other situations, personal information, including personal health information, may need to be disclosed by practice staff in a timely fashion, even if the person's consent has not been obtained. Those members of the practice entitled to disclose personal information in an emergency will be designated, and no other staff member will disclose in such circumstances without gaining authorisation from a designated team member.

In some emergency circumstances, the designated staff of the practice or those acting on their behalf, can – and in some cases must – disclose information that would normally be protected by Ontario's access to information and privacy laws.

PHIPA protects the practice staff from damages, provided that the custodian or head has acted in good faith.Listed below are some circumstances under which the designated practice members may disclose personal information or personal health information, in the absence of an individual's consent.

- *Public Interest and Grave Hazards* If there are reasonable and probable grounds to believe it is in the public interest to do so, and the record of information reveals a grave environmental, health or safety hazard to the public, the designated staff are required to disclose records to the public or to affected persons. This disclosure is required even if the information in the record relates to an individual and may affect his or her interests.

- *Health and Safety of an Individual/ Risk of Serious Harm to Person or Group* When there are compelling circumstances affecting the health and safety of an individual, heads of institutions may disclose personal information to a person other than the individual to whom it relates. Legislation allow this discretionary disclosure.

Where possible the practice will provide the appropriate notice to the individual to whom the information relates. The person may then respond and argue against disclosure. In an emergency, however, it may not be practicable to provide notice in advance of the disclosure.

Similarly, if a health information custodian believes on reasonable grounds that it is necessary, in order to eliminate or reduce a significant risk of serious bodily harm to a person or group of persons, to disclose personal health information without consent, the disclosure may be made.

Such circumstances would even override an individual's prior express instructions not to disclose the relevant personal health information.

- *Disclosures to Public Health Authorities* When an practice health care professional has a legal duty to disclose personal health information, they will do so in accordance with *PHIPA*, which also permits them to disclose personal health information without a patient's consent to the Chief Medical Officer of Health or to a local medical officer of health, in order to comply with the purpose of the *health protection legislation*. That purpose includes preventing the spread of disease, and promoting and protecting the health of the people of Ontario.

- *Compassionate disclosure.* In situations calling for compassion, when there is a need to notify the next of kin or a friend about an individual who is injured, ill or deceased, the practice may disclose personal information or personal health information without consent in order to facilitate this contact.

Similarly, a practice health care professional may also disclose personal health information about a person who is deceased for the purpose of informing any person who it is reasonable to inform that the individual is deceased and the circumstances of his or her death.

An practice health care professional may also disclose personal health information about a deceased person or a person suspected to be deceased (cause of death, or identifying information, for example) to his or her spouse, partner, sibling or child if it is reasonably required to enable these persons to make decisions about their own health care or about the health care of their children.

- *.Health care purpose* When consent cannot be obtained in a timely manner and disclosure is reasonably necessary for the provision of health care, an practice health care professional may disclose personal health information to certain other health information custodians (unless a person has pro-actively forbidden disclosure of the relevant personal health information).

Responsibility of practice health care professionals

The practice health care professionals will seek to protect patient privacy at all times.

They will follow this code of conduct and act in accordance with relevant legislation.

Where there is reasonable doubt, they will seek the guidance of a colleague.

Where this cannot resolve an uncertainty, they will seek the advice of the Information and Privacy Commissioner or an authorised delegated authority.

Table 32 Sample privacy policy for dentists in Ontario

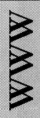

Web link

There is a link provided to the major Canadian provincial dental associations on the web site to help with provincial privacy issues

☑ Exercise 8

Consider your own practice. Identify key categories of information. How long do you retain each type of information?

Information category	Retention time

Think Box

Before we leave this chapter, think about the following question:

Having read about the guidance in your jurisdiction: how confident are you that you are operating within the law?

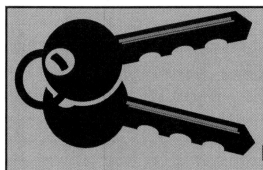

Key points from this chapter

This chapter is all derived from the five basic principles:

1. Don't use patient information unless absolutely necessary.

2. Use the minimum necessary.

3. Access on a strict need-to-know basis.

4. Be aware of responsibilities.

5. Understand and comply with the law.

Chapter 7 Keeping your patients' data safe

Once we accept that as clinicians we have a professional duty to protect patient information, it becomes a duty to assess and manage risks arising from the way that we process and store that data.

The increased use of information technology conforms to Gillies' three rules of risk management:

Gillies' Three Rules of Risk Management

The bad news

The more the use technology, the greater the risks associated with its use

The good news

The technology provides tools and methods to manage and reduce the risk, which if used properly can reduce the overall level of risk

What it means

You have a professional responsibility to use the tools provided to reduce the level of risk to the minimum that is reasonably possible

---

Table 33 Gillies' Three Rules of Risk Management

Electronic data faces a different range of risks from paper-based data. In general, it is less at risk from accidental loss, damage or wear and tear. The technology itself can also help to protect the patients' information if used correctly. On the other hand, there are new and different threats to electronic data.

You should consider how to protect your patients' information against:

- *accidental damage*, risks associated with actions which inadvertently lead to damage to the patient information

- *deliberate damage*, risks associated with actions which knowingly lead to damage to the patient information

- *inherent risks*, risks inherent in the use of that particular type of information system.

- *risks due to errors*, risks arising from potential incorrect use of that particular type of information system.

- *risks due to ignorance*, risks arising from a lack of knowledge concerning the particular type of information system *and*

- *opportunity risks*, risks of lost opportunities arising from the nature of the type of information system used.

Some necessary actions will not be your job, but many risks can be reduced by good habits. The following table shows how risk changes as the records systems moves from paper to a local computer system to a system connected to external computer networks.

Risk	Paper	Computerised	Linked
Accidental damage	• Records filed incorrectly and lost • Records destroyed by fire • Records destroyed by flood	• Files deleted in error • System destroyed by fire • System destroyed by flood	• Files deleted in error • System destroyed by fire • System destroyed by flood • Physical damage to communication links
Deliberate damage	• Records stolen • Records by arson	• System stolen • System destroyed by arson	• System stolen • System destroyed by arson • Deliberate damage to communication links
Inherent risks	• Records physically deteriorating due to age	• Threat from viruses • Threat from Year 2000 problem	• Threat from viruses • Threat from Year 2000 problem • Threat from external access ('hacking')
Risks due to errors	• Transcription errors • Errors in assigning Read codes	• Data input errors • Errors due to bugs in computer system	• Data input errors • Errors due to bugs in computer system • Errors due to problems with external communication systems

Risks due to ignorance	• Failure to detect information through ignorance of record contents	• Lack of knowledge re system • Integrity problems due to failure to implement common coding standards within practice • Failure to fully implement strategies to minimise other forms of risk	• Lack of Knowledge re system • Integrity problems due to failure to implement common coding standards within and without practice • Failure to fully implement strategies to minimise other forms of risk
Opportunity risks	• Difficult to get information for health promotion • Difficult to get management information • Difficult to implement coding	• Failure to reduce risk data integrity problems through electronic communications • Human and financial resources devoted to running the system	• Even greater human and financial resources devoted to running the system

Table 34 Summary of risks identified within risk analysis matrix

Risk 1: Protecting your patients information against accidental damage

Paper-based records have always been at risk of accidental damage through the threats of fire and flood. Additional risks include loss due to incorrect filing.

Each of these risks has a corresponding risk for computerised records. Computers can be destroyed by fire or flood or even in extremis cups of coffee! Similarly, records may be filed under a wrong name or deleted accidentally. It is much easier to delete a computerised record accidentally than throw away a physical record accidentally.

Computers have additional risks due to their need for an external power supply, and their technological complexity. Clinical coding makes incorrect data entry potentially more likely, as different clinicians may wish to use different codes for the same condition.

However, the most significant difference is that the technology can provide a means of managing the risks. As we have a duty to keep patient information secure, so there is a duty to make best use of technology to protect the information from accidental damage. The following table shows how we can protect against the identified risks:

Risk	Management
Flood	Regular backups Remote storage of backups
Fire	Regular backups Remote storage of backups
Power failure	Continuous power supply Regular backups
Equipment failure	Regular backups
Incorrect data entry	Data validation Data entry protocols
Accidental deletion of files	Confirmation dialog boxes

Table 35 Managing the risk

A good backup strategy is essential. A typical strategy might look like:

Day	Task
Monday	Incremental backup
Tuesday	Full backup
Wednesday	Incremental backup
Thursday	Incremental backup
Friday	Full backup removed to remote secure destination
Saturday	Incremental backup
Sunday	Incremental backup

Table 36 A backup strategy

Using this schedule gives you daily protection against equipment failure or a power supply failure that beats your power supply backup, or against accidental deletion. It means that you are never more than a week away from full data in the event of a major catastrophe.

Procedures to make backup up copies of the patient record system must be:

- Appropriately planned to ensure that a valid recent copy can be recovered;
- Regularly, correctly and consistently carried out;
- Verified by checking the integrity of the backed up data (on every occasion).

Used backup disks and tapes should be replaced with new media at regular intervals taking account of the manufacturers recommendations on the anticipated working life of the media used. Old backup media should be re-formatted or physically disrupted so as to render any data on them unrecoverable. If the backup procedure offers a choice of backing up different parts of the system, the routine backup procedure should always include a backup of the audit trail.

The organisation should have a policy on data entry to minimise risks in this area. The policy may allow another person to make entries in the patient records on behalf of the responsible healthcare professional. The information on which such entries are based may be a written note, a dictated message or a verbal report by the healthcare professional responsible for the observations or interventions recorded.

Entries made in this way must be:

- transcribed to the computerised record by an authorised trained person who ascribes the entries to the healthcare professional who wrote or dictated the notes;
- monitored in accordance with the practice policy on data entry to ensure the accuracy and correct attribution of the entries made.

The practice system should record details of who, what and when, in an audit trail. Audit trails should be capable of detecting tampering and should be secured against deletion. If reports and correspondence are received electronically from outside the practice, the practice policy should include procedures to ensure that:

- all information received is seen by the person responsible for the original request or by another dentist acting on his or her behalf;
- the information received is filed in the computerised record of the patient to whom it relates.

Finally, confirmatory dialog boxes are an essential part of any system design. They seek to stop you accidentally doing something with unforeseen consequences.

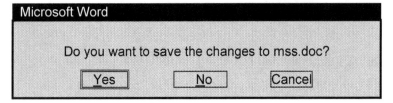

Figure 3 A "Have you lost your presence of mind?" dialog box

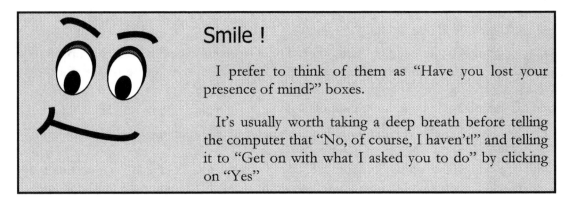

Smile !

I prefer to think of them as "Have you lost your presence of mind?" boxes.

It's usually worth taking a deep breath before telling the computer that "No, of course, I haven't!" and telling it to "Get on with what I asked you to do" by clicking on "Yes"

Risk 2: Protecting your patients information against malicious damage

Electronic records are at risk not just from people who want to read them, but people who thinks it's fun to see if they can.

Paper-based records have always been at risk of unauthorised access. In order to obtain access, however, the interloper has had to be in the presence of the records. Now with the advent of computer networks, people seeking unauthorised access can do so remotely. What is more, some people do it just for fun.

The first line of defence against unauthorised access is physical protection.

Passwords: how good is yours?

Passwords should be longer than 6 characters and use a mixture of letters and numbers to make them as difficult to guess as possible. A truly random combination of 5 letters offers more than 10^{169} combinations, and including numbers increases this to 10^{186} combinations. This is increased further if you mix case. However, as we find it difficult to remember a random sequence we tend to use our pet dog's name or similar!

The other good practice is to change passwords regularly - and always if you suspect that it may be at risk.

Table 37 How good is your password?

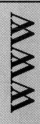

Web link

There is a link provided to a Microsoft facility to test the security of your favourite password from the website accompanying the book.

The UK Department of Health code of conduct offers the following advice.

UK Department of Health advice on physical protection

For all types of records, staff working in offices where records may be seen must:

- Shut/lock doors and cabinets as required.
- Wear building passes/ID if issued.
- Query the status of strangers
- Know who to tell if anything suspicious or worrying is noted.
- Not tell unauthorised personnel how the security systems operate.
- Not breach security themselves.

Manual records must be:

- Formally booked out from their normal filing system.
- Tracked if transferred, with a note made or sent to the filing location of the transfer.
- Returned to the filing location as soon as possible after use.
- Stored securely within the clinic or office, arranged so that the record can be found easily if needed urgently.
- Stored closed when not in use so that contents are not seen accidentally.
- Inaccessible to members of the public and not left even for short periods where they might be looked at by unauthorised persons.
- Held in secure storage with clear labelling. Protective 'wrappers' indicating sensitivity - though not indicating the reason for sensitivity - and permitted access, and the availability of secure means of destruction, eg shredding, are essential.

Table 38 UK Department of Health advice on physical protection

Electronic records add another set of responsibilities, it is important that all staff understand the additional responsibilities that electronic records bring.

UK Department of Health advice on protecting electronic records

- Always log-out of any computer system or application when work on it is finished.

- Don't leave a terminal unattended and logged-in.

- Don't share logins with other people. If other staff have need to access records, then appropriate access should be organised for them - this must not be by using others' access identities.

- Don't reveal passwords to others.

- Change passwords at regular intervals to prevent anyone else using them.

- Avoid using short passwords , or using names or words that are known to be associated with them (eg children's or pet names or birthdays).

- Always clear the screen of a previous patient's information before seeing another.

- Use a password-protected screen-saver to prevent casual viewing of patient information by others.

Table 39 UK Department of Health advice on protecting electronic records

Paper-based records have always been at risk of physical damage. Fire and flood may be initiated deliberately.

Computers are attractive objects in themselves, both to thieves and also to people who write viruses to attack computers. In Salford, Greater Manchester, in the mid-1990s, one practice was so worried about theft from premises, that their entire computer system had to fit onto one laptop that could be removed at night.

Generally, however, whilst physical security is certainly an issue, the threat from viruses is a greater risk. In recent years, the NHSNet has been attacked and breached by the 'I love you' virus, and the Blaster worm.

The following advice is given to general medical practices[7], but applies equally to general dental practices

- Disks received from outside the practice should be checked for viruses by effective and regularly updated anti-virus programmes;

- Files received from outside the practice by electronic transfer should also be checked for viruses.

Every health care organisation should have a security policy that takes full account of the need for confidentiality as well as authentication and integrity of the computerised patient record system. The security policy should take account of local circumstances and risks but should specifically address the points under the headings below:

- Security policy

- Security organization

- Asset classification and control

- Personnel security

- Physical and environmental security

- Communications and operations management

- Access control

- System development and maintenance

- Business continuity management

- Compliance

The policy should recognise the need for data entry to be restricted to properly trained and authorised people. It must take full account of the need for entries to be accurate, complete and attributed to the person responsible for the observations or interventions recorded. When considering the issue of authentication, all staff should be aware that they may be held liable for the content and accuracy of information that appears to have been entered by them or on their behalf. It is therefore important that the security features of the system and procedures followed by the practice combine to

---

[7] *Source: Good Practice Guidelines for General Practice Electronic Patient Records*
The Joint Computing Group of the General Practitioners' Committee and the Royal College of General Practitioners

minimise the risk of a record entry being accidentally or fraudulently attributed to the wrong user.

It may be necessary to prove that an entry was or was not made by the person to whom it is attributed. This means that, since most record entries are logged as being the responsibility of the individual whose password is currently entered, it should never be acceptable for an entry to be made into a record when someone else has logged into the system. More generally, it is essential that all users:

- have a unique user identity and password;

- keep their password secret and do not divulge it to other users for any reason;

- change their passwords at frequent intervals;

- log out of workstations when their task at that workstation is finished and never leave a workstation logged in but unattended.

The policy should ensure that the organisation has a clearly laid out disaster recovery plan. This will need to address the temporary replacement of the organisation's electronic functions with paper-based alternatives, the retention and subsequent entry of these temporary records into the electronic record system when it becomes available again and the extraction of essential information from ancillary systems such as any electronic appointment book's backup.

So much for protecting your patients' records. What if your patient wants to see their own record?

What the UK Information Commissioner said about patients' rights to see their records

The Data Protection Act 1998 was implemented on 1 March 2000. Although there are periods of transitional relief during which certain provisions of the new legislation need not be complied with, the implementation of the new legislation will have an immediate impact in respect of subject access to health records.

The right of subject access allows the individual to gain access to personal data of which he is the subject. Typically this will involve supplying an individual with copies of records relating to him when asked to do so. For general information about the right of subject access see 'The Data Protection Act 1998 - An Introduction'.

A 'health record' is defined in the 1998 Act as being any record which consists of information relating to the physical or mental health or condition of an individual, and has been made by or on behalf of a health professional in connection with the care of that individual.

The definition of a 'health record' could apply to material held on an X-ray or an MRI scan, for example. This means that when a subject access request is made, the information contained in such material must be supplied to the applicant within the fee structure described below. It is clear, therefore, that many of the records being held by NHS Trusts, surgeries and other health care institutions will constitute 'health records' and will therefore fall within the scope of the 1998 Act's subject access provisions.

What about the Access to Health Records Act 1990?

This piece of legislation formerly gave individuals a right of access to manual health records - ie to the sort of non-automated records that the Data Protection Act 1984 did not apply to. However, the Access to Health Records Act 1990 has now been repealed except for the sections dealing with requests for access to records relating to the deceased. Requests for access to records relating to the deceased will continue to be made under the Access to Health Records Act 1990. However, requests for access to health records relating to living individuals, whether the records are manual or automated, will now fall within the scope of the Data Protection Act 1998's subject access provisions and must be dealt with in the manner stipulated in that Act.

How much can be charged for granting subject access?

A maximum fee of £10 may be charged for granting subject access to health records that are being automatically processed, or that are recorded with the intention that they be so processed. In effect, this means that only £10 may be charged for granting access to the sort of records that the Data Protection Act 1984 applied to.

A maximum fee of £50 may be charged for granting subject access to manual records, or to a mixture of manual and automated records, where the request for subject access will be granted by supplying a copy of the information in permanent form. It should be noted that there is no express provision for any fee to be charged for copying or despatching copies of records. However, the £50 chargeable fee will allow for some of the costs incurred by granting subject access to be recovered.

No fee may be charged where the subject access request is to be complied with other than by supplying a copy of the information in a permanent form - ie by allowing the applicant to inspect the record. This provision only relates to requests for access to non-automated records at least some of which was made after the beginning of the period of 40 days immediately preceding the date of the request. This provision broadly replicates the provision of the Access to Health Records Act 1990 that, in effect, allows patients to look at recently created records for free.

The fee for granting subject access to manual health records had been due to reduce to £10 on 24 October 2001. The higher fee was originally by way of transitional relief, allowing for the fact that under the Access to Health Records Act 1990, (whose substantive provisions were incorporated into the Data Protection Act 1998), much higher fees could be charged. However, the government announced on 27 September 2001 that the £50 fee would continue 'for the time being'. This means that data controllers can continue to charge a maximum fee of up to £50 where a copy of the information contained in manual health records is provided in a permanent form. This continuation is provided for in The Data Protection (Subject Access) (Fees and Miscellaneous Provisions) (Amendment) Regulations 2001. It was also stated that the Government is committed to continuing discussions with key interest groups and to working closely with the Information Commissioner with the aim of achieving a long-term solution.

You may be required to provide a description of the data; a description of the purpose/s for which the data are being or are to be processed; a description of the recipients or classes or recipients of the data - ie persons to whom the data are disclosed

The data subject must also be given; any information available to the controller as to the source of the data and an explanation as to how any automated decision taken about the data subject has been made.

Table 40 What the UK Information Commissioner said about patients' rights to see their records

Risk 3: Protecting your patients information against inherent risks

Since paper-based systems are very simple compared to computer systems, inherent risks are also limited. The greatest risk inherent in a paper-based system is deterioration in paper and ink over a long period of time.

By comparison, computer systems carry much greater risk. The systems themselves carry a significant risk of mechanical breakdown, particularly in critical components such as hard disks. Since computers are dependent upon a continuous power supply, they are at risk from an interruption to the electrical power supply, either internal to the practice or externally.

In addition, computer systems face inherent risks in a number of high profile areas. Computer are threatened by viruses, programmes designed to infiltrate computer systems and then to cause damage once in place. Whilst the risk has probably been overstated, the potential damage can be severe and prevention strategies need to be adopted.

Linked systems face the additional inherent problem of 'hacking', or unauthorised external access. Any external connection to the Health Authority, Internet or NHSNet is a potential risk. This may again be minimised by correct procedure, although, in the case of NHSNet, this may be beyond the control of the practice concerned.

Risk 4: Protecting your patients information against risks due to errors

The most common form of errors in paper based systems are transcription errors. 33% of paper based records may contain errors.[8],[9] However, fortunately, many of these are not

---

[8] *Wyatt, J.C. (1994) Clinical data systems, part 1: data and mechanical records, Lancet 344, 1543-1547.*

in critical information, representing spelling errors in name and address information for example. Procedures can exacerbate this problem by placing extra steps in the data input process.

Comparable errors can be found in computer based records. Wyatt identifies this as the key risk in clinical data systems. Good system design and the use of predetermined option selection from a menu as opposed to free text entry can be used to reduce error rates. This can be particularly helpful in reducing error rates in non-intuitive data such as Read codes. However, faults in software can also introduce additional errors. Left unmanaged, this can give rise to even greater error rates, with error rates of over 50% being reported [10,11]

Similarly, in connected systems, external corruption of data transfer can introduce errors.

Risk 5: Protecting your patients information against risks due to ignorance

Paper based records systems do not facilitate the detection of information within them. Therefore, users can be ignorant of the content of the records themselves. Although computers can facilitate the finding of specific information, they can also increase the risk of problems caused by ignorance.

Users of computer based systems require knowledge of the systems themselves and ignorance of this can lead to erroneous results or a waste of resources in terms of time. Data integrity problems can be caused by ignorance of the need to implement a common coding policy across a practice. Whilst not exclusively associated with computerised practices, coding is often only implemented after computerisation. Linked practices increase this risk by requiring a common coding policy across all organisational units connected by the system.

Ignorance of strategies to reduce all forms of risk associated with computer systems in itself presents a risk as using a computerised system without strategies for risk reduction does significantly increase risk for all the reasons outlined above.

Risk 6: Protecting your patients information against opportunity risks

The risk of lost opportunities within paper based systems is very high. It is difficult to extract information for health promotion and for monitoring, evaluation and audit. It is difficult to implement a coding policy. Finally, it is difficult to spot any anomalous trends that may exist within a paper-based dataset.

---

[9] *McKee, M. Routine data: a resource for clinical audit? Quality in Health Care, 2, 104-111*

[10] *Dixon, J. (1994) NW Thames Small Area Analysis Project: Phase 2 Data accuracy Study, London School of Hygiene and Tropical Medicine.*

[11] *Smith, M.F. (1995) New computer system paradigm needed for clinical information systems, Proceedings of the European Conference on Health Informatics, Paris, 143-9, ISBN 0 906694 49 3.*

The opportunity risks associated with running an isolated computer system are the failure to maximise data integrity through the use of electronic communications. Further, there is an opportunity risk associated with the human and financial resources associated with running the system itself.

For connected systems, the opportunity risk associated with data integrity is reduced but the greater resources required raise that particular opportunity risk.

Sample practices

These studies are based upon actual practices known to the author, and taken from various time periods. They are anonymised for the purpose of confidentiality.

Sample 1   A paper-based practice

This practice has no computer system. Their activity is all private, some with a major dental plan, the rest funded directly by patients.

It has managed with a card-based system thus far because of its small size. However, it is planned to install a system that will be connected to the . Currently, the patient records and other data is kept on card indexes. The implications of this are much greater time spent on filing and recording patient information than computerised practices that are comparable in size. More significant perhaps is the potential for error and the difficulty of spotting errors. Experience in other practices have revealed a discrepancy rate of 5 to 10% between paper recording systems and the insurance company's central records.

The risks

This practice represents a classic paper based practice. It faces all the risks identified in the matrix. The practice themselves have identified the problems, and hence the plan to move to a computer based system. However, the move to a connected computer based system will involve many new risks that must be managed effectively.

Sample 2   A computerised practice Three dentists, 5,000 patients

The practice

This inner city practice provides publicly funded dentistry to a deprived area within a large conurbation. It has a computer system based around a single machine. Many of the characteristics of this practice arose from its inner city location:

- Due to high levels of crime in the area, it was felt that the computer could not be left in the surgery overnight. As a consequence the system was based upon a laptop machine shared by all the staff.

- The practice was characterised by a high level of patient and staff turnover

The use of a single laptop meant that staff had limited access to the computer. The absence of formal training for staff arriving since the adoption of the system five years previously had compounded this inexperience and led to a considerable lack of confidence amongst the administrative staff in the use of the computer. This problem was made worse by the existence of a branch surgery where all data was recorded on paper, transferred physically to the main surgery and then entered onto the computer.

These factors led to very limited use of the computer system and a dependence upon the local primary care trust for certain information, Experience elsewhere suggests that this dependence is undesirable unless there are strong links between the dentists own computer systems and those of the local Trust. This was clearly not the case here.

The system was also not used for compiling practice reports, which again causes duplication of work and introduces the possibility of data transcription errors.

The personnel interviewed, both the dentist and his staff, felt that these problems were exacerbated by poor documentation, poor training and unnecessary complexity of the computer processes.

The risks

This practice highlights how computerisation can increase risk dramatically. The most obvious example is the risk of the computer being stolen. This has in turn led to the adoption of a very limited computer based solution, which has specific risks attached to it.

The dependency upon the local primary care trust has major risks associated with it in terms of data integrity. The problems with access and training increases risks due to ignorance and highlights many opportunity risks which are normally associated with paper based systems, there are risks of information not being available for health promotion, management and monitoring.

Sample 3   A connected practice: One-dentist, 1200 patients

The practice

This practice had a well-established computer system and the dentist and his practice manager were very comfortable with the technology. Extensive use of the computer system was made for preventative treatment through screening and routine recall programs. The system used was a multi-user system with terminals in the reception area, consulting room and practice manager's office. System maintenance and housekeeping was carried out by the practice manager, although the dentist was obviously highly computer literate. The system was used for all patient records, prescribing screening and compiling practice reports. The system was used to send out SMS messages as reminders of appointments where patients had given permission for this to happen.

Direct links to the two main insurance providers were used for reporting purposes. Confidentiality issues were a high priority and a mailbox system was under discussion to prevent the insurance company from having general access to the system.

The biggest problem highlighted in getting to this point had been the transfer from manual to computer patient records. Apart from the issue of the amount of time involved, the quality of information was considered critical. 33% of paper-based records showed inconsistencies, eg members of the same household were listed as living at different addresses. As a result, the input of patient data was handled by the dentist himself, in order to preserve as far as possible the integrity of the data.

The risks

This practice highlights how a well-organised practice can adopt strategies to manage and actively reduce risks. The process of computerisation was used to actively reduce the risk of data integrity errors from the original paper system. The additional risks associated with linkage are well understood and managed.

The overall effect of computerisation is that the risk to information integrity within the practice has been significantly reduced through the well-managed introduction of a connected computerised system.

Freedom of information

The UK Freedom of Information Act only applies to public authorities, including NHS Trusts, and companies that are wholly owned by public authorities.

UK dentists I have spoken to are unclear whether the Act applies to them.

The Freedom of Information Act applies to any dental practice that undertakes any NHS activity at all. For dentists with no public activity, the Freedom of Information Act provides a model of good practice

Practices covered by the Act are obliged to provide information:

- Through a Publication Scheme

- In response to requests made under the general right of access.

A Publication Scheme is both a public commitment to make certain information available and a guide to how that information can be obtained. All publication schemes have to be approved by the Information Commissioner and should be reviewed by authorities periodically to ensure they are accurate and up to date.

When responding to requests, there are set procedures that public authorities need to follow. These procedures include:

- The time public authorities are allowed for responding to requests. In general, organisations have 20 working days to respond to requests.
- The fees or amount that public authorities can charge for dealing with requests. Public authorities are not obliged to deal with requests if the costs of finding the information exceeds a set amount known as the appropriate limit.
- Public authorities need not comply with vexatious or repeated requests.

The Act also recognises that there are valid reasons for withholding information by setting out a number of exemptions from right to know.

It is important to remember that the Freedom of Information Act does not require organisations to reveal personal data in breach of the Data Protection Act and if an individual clinician working within the NHS receives a request under the Freedom of information Act, they should refer it to their Caldicott Guardian or Information Governance Lead.

In the United States, there are a number of individual pieces of freedom of information legislation, as well as a number of other sunshine laws intended to increase the openness and transparency of government. The most significant piece of legislation is the federal Freedom of Information Act

Specific legislation may require that all government meetings be open to the public, or that written records be released upon request. The usual intent of these laws is to enable citizens and journalists to examine government activity to detect political corruption, or to allow them to have input into government decisions that affect them. Many consider strong laws guaranteeing freedom of information to be vitally important to journalism. However, as dentistry in North America has remained outside the public sector, it has not been affected by public freedom of information legislation.

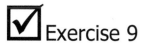Exercise 9

Consider your own practice. How often do you back up your data?

Backup category	Frequency
Local incremental backup	
Local complete backup	
Remote complete backup	

Think Box

Before we leave this chapter, think about the following question:

Having read about the guidance in your jurisdiction: how confident are you that your data is safe against the threats of accidental damage, unauthorised access and malicious damage?

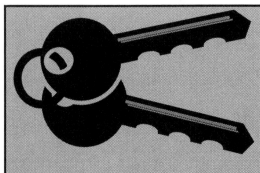

Key points from this chapter

Your data is at risk from

- Accidental damage
- Unauthorised access
- Malicious damage

You have a responsibility to proactively protect your patient data from these risks.

If you have any interaction with the UK NHS, you must take account of the freedom of information legislation for public bodies

Chapter 8 Some things that might just make it all worthwhile for you

Informatics can help you find information

Informatics is not just about helping patients, it can help you do your job, or develop your knowledge and skills. As a dental professional, you have a professional obligation to ensure that your knowledge is up to date.

There is a huge amount of information available to you, and you can use the technology to help you find what you need. Generally, you need to use one set of resources to find what is available, and another to actually access the material.

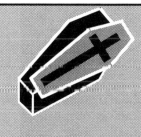

Zombie warning

There is a popular perception that if information is on the Internet, it is not reliable. For that matter, the popular perception that a randomised control trial published in a major journal is Gospel truth.

In reality, these days, most traditional academic sources of evidence can be accessed on-line, sometimes by payment of a fee, although often if you work within the UK NHS, they may have paid this on your behalf.

Resources to help you find information

On the Internet, you will find a range of tools to help you find the information you need. These are often characterised in two types:

- Internet search engines. These are tools that search the Internet for information. Examples would be Google, Ask, and AltaVista. There are also engines that Dogpile which combine results from several search engines

- Bibliographic databases. These are tools that search the academic literature for peer reviewed articles. They are usually linked to a particular clinical community, eg MEDLINE is used to search the medical literature, CINAHL to search the nursing literature.

Let us suppose that you wish to find information about tooth decay in children. If you go to the Internet and go to http://www.google.com and enter the search terms:

"tooth decay children":

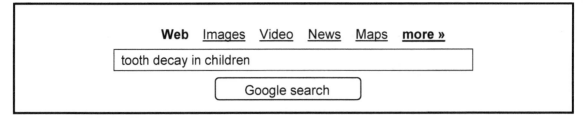

Figure 4 Entering search terms into Google

this is roughly you will see:

BBC - Health - Conditions - **Tooth decay in children**
Causes and affects of **tooth decay** and its treatment.
www.bbc.co.uk/health/conditions/**toothdecay**2.shtml - 37k - <u>Cached</u> - <u>Similar pages</u>

Tooth decay: What problems can **children** experience with cavities?
Suggestions for minimizing the risk of **tooth decay in children**.
www.animated-teeth.com/**tooth_decay**/t5_**tooth_decay_children**.htm - 20k - <u>Cached</u> - <u>Similar pages</u>

What is **tooth decay**?
The formation of **tooth decay** ("cavities") can be a significant problem for some individuals, either as **children** or adults. **Tooth decay** can, however, ...
www.animated-teeth.com/**tooth_decay**/t1_**tooth_decay**_cavities.htm - 19k - <u>Cached</u> - <u>Similar pages</u>

ADA.org: Oral Health Topics: Early Childhood **Tooth Decay (Baby ...**
This page provides current information about Early Childhood **Tooth Decay** (Baby ... a Caries-Risk Assessment Tool (CAT) for Infants, **Children** and Adolescents ...
www.ada.org/public/topics/**decay**_childhood.asp - 37k - <u>Cached</u> - <u>Similar pages</u>

Child dental hygiene, caring for teeth & **tooth decay in children**
BUPA health fact sheet - information for parents on child dental hygiene including diet, caring for teeth and **tooth decay in children**, with advice on taking ...
hcd2.bupa.co.uk/fact_sheets/html/child_dental.html - 43k - <u>Cached</u> - <u>Similar pages</u>

Figure 5 Results from Google

This window shows you two types of information. The left hand column provides the actual results of the search. The information at the top and down the right hand side is provided by people who have paid Google to put it there.

One of the common complaints from searchers outside of the US is that the results are very US-centric. You can fix this by using your national Google only to look for your own country results (eg select "pages from the UK") or any other country for that matter:

<table>
<tr><td>

BBC - Health - Conditions - **Tooth decay in children**
Causes and affects of **tooth decay** and its treatment.
www.bbc.co.uk/health/conditions/**toothdecay**2.shtml - 37k
- Cached - Similar pages

Child dental hygiene, caring for teeth & **tooth decay in children**
BUPA health fact sheet - information for parents on child dental hygiene including diet, caring for teeth and **tooth decay in children**, with advice on taking ...
hcd2.bupa.co.uk/fact_sheets/html/child_dental.html - 43k -
Cached - Similar pages

British Dental Health Foundation
Toothache is painful and upsetting, especially in **children**, and the main cause is still **tooth decay**. This is due to too much sugar, too often, in the diet. ...
www.dentalhealth.org.uk/faqs/leafletdetail.php?LeafletID=3
- 24k - Cached - Similar pages

Tooth decay: What problems can **children** experience with cavities?
Suggestions for minimizing the risk of **tooth decay in children**.
www.animated-
teeth.com/**tooth_decay**/t5_**tooth_decay_children**.htm -
20k - Cached - Similar pages

What is **tooth decay**?
The formation of **tooth decay** ("cavities") can be a significant problem for some individuals, either as **children** or adults. **Tooth decay** can, however, ...
www.animated-
teeth.com/**tooth_decay**/t1_**tooth_decay**_cavities.htm -
19k - Cached - Similar pages

</td><td>

Sponsored Links

Dentist **Children**
Free Dentist **Children** info
Find what you're looking for!
www.dental-101.com

Tooth decay
Find the right answers about **tooth decay**.
www.healthline.com

Tooth Decay In Children
Connect with Others Talk about **Tooth Decay In Children** & more!
www.myLot.cc

Tooth Decay In Children
All you need to know about **Tooth Decay In Children**
dentist.freesourcenow.com

</td></tr>
</table>

Figure 6 British results from Google, including Sponsored links

This information may be extremely helpful if you are looking for information for patients, for example, to find the nearest self help group, or to provide good advice on managing chronic conditions. However, it is unlikely to lead you to the most up to date evidence in the research literature.

This may be accessed through the bibliographic databases such as MEDLINE, which is hosted by the National Library of Medicine in Washington DC. There is no internationally recognised database specifically for dentistry, but many of them have literature relevant to dentistry.

Common bibliographic databases that you might wish to access include:

Database	Contents
Medline	Abstracts from the medical literature
Cinahl	Abstracts from the nursing literature
Psycinfo	Abstracts from the psychological literature
Embase	Index of the world's literature on human medicine and related disciplines.
AMED	Abstracts from the Allied and Complementary Medicine literature
British Nursing Index	Index of the British nursing literature
DH-Data	Abstracts regarding health service and hospital administration; also medical toxicology and environmental health
Zetoc	British Library Electronic Table of Contents (ETOC) database
Images MD	50000 high-quality images spanning all of internal medicine

Table 41 Bibliographic databases. They usually produce abstracts, not full text

Although these databases will provide access to a huge range of articles, they generally only list the abstracts. You will need another source for the article themselves. Happily, the National Library for Health can help here too.

MEDLINE may be accessed through a range of portals. PubMed is may not be the best, but is available free on the Internet.

CINAHL is not available free on the web, but may be accessed through a University or health library. See below for more information.

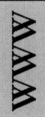

Web link

There are links provided to many of the resources, bibliographic databases and search engines via the web site accompanying the book

Type http://www.nlm.nih.gov into your internet browser:

Health Information	**Especially for:**	**List of NLM▶▶ Databases and Resources**
Library Catalog & Services	● The Public	
History of Medicine	● Health Care Professionals	**PubMed**
Online Exhibitions & Digital Projects	● Researchers	Biomedical journal literature from MEDLINE/PubMed
	● Librarians	
Human Genome Resources	● Publishers	**MedlinePlus**
Biomedical Research & Informatics	**Current Health News**	Health and drug information for patients, family and friends
Environmental Health & Toxicology	A Drink May Help High Blood Pressure Risk (01/03/07)	
Health Services Research & Public Health	Down Syndrome Screening Recommended for All Expectant Moms (01/03/07)	**Household Products Database**
Health Information Technology	Patients' Lost Time Boosts Cost of Cancer Care (01/03/07)	Health and safety information on household products
About the National Library of Medicine	More Health News	
Grants & Funding	**NLM News and Press Releases**	**NLM Gateway**
Training & Outreach	NLM Announces the New Bioethics Information Resources Web Page (12/18/06)	Simultaneous searching in 20 NLM databases
Network of Medical Libraries	"Dream Anatomy" catalogue published (12/14/06)	
	NLM Consultants Honored (12/12/06)	
	NIH Launches dbGaP, a Database of Genome Wide Association Studies (12/12/06)	

Figure 7 The US National library of Medicine

Click on the Visit Site button in the PubMed section:

Now if we enter our search terms here and click on "Go" we get a different kind of result. MEDLINE produces a list of articles but only provides us with access to the abstracts in most cases.

Items 1 - 20 of 11796   Page 1 of 590   Next

1: Marshall TA, Eichenberger-Gilmore JM, Larson MA, Warren JJ, Levy SM.   Related Articles
 Comparison of the intakes of sugars by young children with and without dental caries experience.
J Am Dent Assoc. 2007 Jan;138(1):39-46.
PMID: 17197400 [PubMed - as supplied by publisher]
2: Elias-Boneta AR, Psoter W, Elias-Viera AE, Jimenez P, Toro C.   Related Articles, Links
 Relationship between dental caries experience (DMFS) and dental fluorosis in 12-year-old Puerto Ricans.
Community Dent Health. 2006 Dec;23(4):244-50.
PMID: 17194073 [PubMed - in process]
3: Schulte AG, Momeni A, Pieper K.   Related Articles, Links
 Caries prevalence in 12-year-old children from Germany. Results of the 2004 national survey.
Community Dent Health. 2006 Dec;23(4):197-202.
PMID: 17194065 [PubMed - in process]
4: Chestnutt IG.   Related Articles, Links
 Chlorhexidine varnish has caries-reducing potential.
Evid Based Dent. 2006;7(4):93.
PMID: 17187036 [PubMed - in process]
5: Zhang Q, van Palenstein Helderman WH, Van't Hof MA, Truin GJ.   Related Articles, Links
 Chlorhexidine varnish for preventing dental caries in children, adolescents and young adults: a systematic review.
Eur J Oral Sci. 2006 Dec;114(6):449-55.
PMID: 17184224 [PubMed - in process]
6: Mohebbi SZ, Virtanen JI, Vahid-Golpayegani M, Vehkalahti MM.   Related Articles, Links
 Early childhood caries and dental plaque among 1-3-year-olds in Tehran, Iran.
J Indian Soc Pedod Prev Dent. 2006 Dec;24(4):177-81.
    PMID: 17183180 [PubMed - in process]

Figure 8 Results from Medline accessed through PubMed.

MEDLINE is generally recognised as something of a gold standard. However, it has a number of limitations:

- It only lists abstracts
- It is U.S. centric, which is fine if you are based there, but not for the rest of the world!
- It is a medical database so may well not serve the needs of other health care professionals, or indeed areas of medicine such as general practice.

Currently, a hybrid type of tool is emerging, which uses internet search techniques to search the academic literature to find information. An example of this would be Google Scholar.

To illustrate how this works consider the same search terms:

Type http://scholar.google.com/ into your Internet browser.

Use "tooth decay children" as your search terms.

The results look like this:

Results **1 - 10** of about **8,270** for <u>tooth</u> <u>decay</u> <u>children</u>. **(0.07** seconds)

All Results

<u>W Loesche</u>

<u>P Caufield</u>

<u>P Domoto</u>

<u>P Weinstein</u>

<u>B Edelstein</u>

Mexican-American parents with children **at risk for baby bottle** tooth decay: **pilot study at a migrant ...** - <u>group of 2 »</u>
P Weinstein, P Domoto, K Wohlers, M Koday - ASDC J Dent Child, 1992 - ncbi.nlm.nih.gov
Mexican-American parents with **children** at risk for baby bottle **tooth decay**: pilot study at a migrant farmworkers clinic. Weinstein **...**
<u>Cited by 26</u> - <u>Related Articles</u> - <u>Web Search</u> - <u>BL Direct</u>

Role of Streptococcus mutans in human dental decay. - <u>group of 7 »</u>
WJ Loesche - Microbiology and Molecular Biology Reviews, 1986 - Am Soc Microbiol
... Dental infections such as **tooth decay** and periodontal disease are perhaps the most common bacterial infections in **... tooth** substance lost to dental **decay** (69). **...**
<u>Cited by 595</u> - <u>Related Articles</u> - <u>Web Search</u>

Parental awareness, habits, and social factors and their relationship to baby bottle tooth decay. <u>group of 2 »</u>
C Febres, EA Echeverri, HJ Keene - Pediatr Dent, 1997 - ncbi.nlm.nih.gov
... parental awareness, habits, and social factors in a particular parent population and the occurrence of baby bottle **tooth decay** (BBTD) in their **children**. **...**
<u>Cited by 19</u> - <u>Related Articles</u> - <u>Web Search</u> - <u>BL Direct</u>

Water fluoridation, poverty and tooth decay **in 12-year-old** children - <u>group of 9 »</u>
CM Jones, H Worthington - Journal of Dentistry, 2000 - Elsevier
... inequalities are reduced. Author Keywords: Water fluoridation; Deprivation; Townsend; **Tooth decay**; DMFT; **Children**; Electoral wards. **...**
<u>Cited by 11</u> - <u>Related Articles</u> - <u>Web Search</u> - <u>BL Direct</u>

Water fluoridation and tooth decay: **Results from the 1986-1987 national survey of US school** children **...**
JA Yiamouyiannis - Fluoride, 1990 - csa.com
Water fluoridation and **tooth decay**: Results from the 1986-1987 national survey of US school **children**. JA Yiamouyiannis Fluoride 23:22, 55-67, 1990. **...**
<u>Cited by 11</u> - <u>Related Articles</u> - <u>Web Search</u>

Figure 9 Results from Google Scholar

Resources to allow you to read the actual evidence you have found

Once you have found the evidence that you need, then you need to be able to gain access to the information itself. This can be done through a range of on-line library facilities, notably the National Library for Health, if you are based in the UK and working with the NHS.

Type http://www.library.nhs.uk into your browser.

National Library for Health

HOME SEARCH RESOURCES NEWS & RSS   MY LIBRARY CLINICAL SUMMARIES CLINICAL Q&A

Figure 10 The UK National Library for Health

RESOURCES

Evidence Based Reviews

Bandolier, Clinical Knowledge Summaries, Cochrane Library, NHS Economic Evaluation Database ...

Guidance

Guidelines Finder, NICE Guidance, NLH Protocols & Care Pathways ...

Specialist Libraries

Collections of the best available evidence for particular specialties...

Books, Journals and Bibliographic Databases

AMED, BioMed Central, British Nursing Index, e-books, Embase, Medline, My Journals, Psycinfo, ...

Images

Images MD

For Patients

Best Treatments, Dipex, NHS Direct Online, Patient.co.uk, ...

Drugs

British National Formulary, British National Formulary for Children, National Electronic Library for Medicines ...

Figure 11 Resources section of The National Library for Health Homepage

The National library for Health provides a huge library of resources available at your desk for those of you working in the UK NHS.

In order to access them, you may need to enter via the NHSNet or use your Athens Password, (if you don't think you have one, contact your local health librarian) to prove that you are an NHS staff member, (if you are!) This is because for many of the resources, the NHS has paid a subscription on your behalf.

As an example of how information technology can provide a much greater service than a paper based solution, it's hard to think of a better one. On the other hand, the sheer quantity of information can be daunting. Your local health librarian is still an invaluable guide even in this electronic age.

Many academic resources are available on-line but require a subscription. However, through the National Library for Health, the NHS has paid most of these charges for you. Therefore, in order to access these resources, you will need to register and use an Athens ID.

You can use the search facility to find resources. For example, here are the results form a search on "oral health"

Guidelines for **oral_health** care for long-stay patients and residents
Publisher: British Society for Disability and Oral Health **Publication Date:** 1 January 2000
Publication Type: Care Guideline
Source: Guidelines Finder

More detail | Full text | Save Result

Guidelines for the development of local standards of **oral_health** care for dependent, dysphagic, critically and terminally-ill patients
Publisher: British Society for Disability and Oral Health **Publication Date:** 1 January 2000
Publication Type: Care Guideline
Source: Guidelines Finder

More detail | Full text | Save Result

Oral_health care for people with mental **health** problems: guidelines and recommendations
Publisher: British Society for Disability and Oral Health **Publication Date:** 1 January 2000
Publication Type: Care Guideline
Source: Guidelines Finder

More detail | Full text | Save Result

Guidelines for **oral_health** care for people with a physical disability
Publisher: British Society for Disability and Oral Health **Publication Date:** 1 January 2000
Publication Type: Care Guideline
Source: Guidelines Finder

More detail | Full text | Save Result

Clinical guidelines and integrated care pathways for the **oral_health** care of people with learning disabilities 2001
Publisher: Royal College of Surgeons of England **Publication Date:** 1 January 2000
Publication Type: Care Guideline
Source: Guidelines Finder

Figure 12 Results on a search on "oral health" in the UK NLH

For dentists, a key resource is the oral health specialist library:

Welcome to the Oral Health Specialist Library

The library aims to encourage the use of evidence in practice and optimum care for all patients by providing rapid access to recent, reliable evidence.

Research is critically appraised and summarised in accordance with our quality policy. We welcome all views and suggestions to ensure that the library is as useful as possible.

The library is aimed primarily to support oral health professionals, trainees and other health care professionals, however, it is also freely available to the general public. We regret that we are unable to respond to personal medical queries and such messages will not be answered. For such matters we would advise you to contact NHS Direct or your usual dentist.

The Specialist Library is being developed by a team based at Cardiff University and guided by a UK wide steering group. More information about the team is available from about us.

What's New

04/12/06

The British Society for Disability and Oral Health Scientific Meeting will be taking place on Friday 8th December in London. The aims of the conference are to review progress with the development of the Specialty in Specialist Care Dentistry. The conference will offer solutions to practical issues relating to patient care, and for the first time will provide an expert panel to respond to members issues. Select here for further details

03/10/06

Five new relevant systematic reviews have been published in Issue 4 of the Cochrane Library:

- Home-based chemically-induced whitening of teeth in adults

- Interventions for replacing missing teeth: dental implants in fresh extraction sockets (immediate, immediate-delayed and delayed implants)

- Orthodontic treatment for deep bite and retroclined upper front teeth in children

- Pit and fissure sealants versus fluoride varnishes for preventing dental caries in children and adolescents

- Slow-release fluoride devices for the control of dental decay

29/09/06

The 2007 IADR EBD Network Systematic Review Prize has recently been announced. The award encourages researchers to conduct the highest quality systematic reviews on important oral health topics. Protocols outlining the methods and timeline for completing the review should be submitted by 30th November 2006. The award will consist of £7,000 to support research activity plus a certificate. Please select this link for further details.

04/08/06

Three new relevant Cochrane systematic reviews have been published in Issue 3 of the Cochrane Library:

- Adhesives for fixed orthodontic bands

- Complete or ultraconservative removal of decayed tissue in unfilled teeth

- Interventions for the prevention and management of oropharyngeal candidiasis associated with HIV infection in adults and children

Two reviews have also been updated:

- Potassium containing toothpastes for dentine hypersensitivity

- Screening programmes for the early detection and prevention of oral cancer

Figure 13 Contents of the specialist oral health library

The oral health library has other useful resources, notably a section outlining the evidential basis for current media stories in dentistry:

Dentistry in the News

Seen a headline in the news regarding oral health and want to know more about it? 'Dentistry in the news' assesses the quality of the original research behind the news headlines, and examines how closely the media have reported it.

Jun 2005	Can fluoride water cause cancer?
Apr 2005	Can mini 'light sabres' replace toothbrushes in battling gum disease?
Mar 2005	Are sports drinks dissolving teeth?
Feb 2005	Can tooth brushing cut heart risk?
Feb 2005	Tooth filling cuts out drill
Jan 2005	Vioxx and coronary heart disease
Nov 2004	Should babies be breastfed to grow straight teeth?
Sept 2004	Is there an effective alternative to dental sedation for children?
Jun 2004	Are childhood lifestyles to blame for bad teeth in adulthood?
Apr 2004	Dental X-ray baby threat
Mar 2004	Are fizzy drinks to blame for bad teeth?
Dec 2003	Is early treatment of buck teeth beneficial?
Jun 2003	Can brushing too hard damage teeth?
May 2003	Does herbal tea damage teeth?
Mar 2003	Can passive smoking cause dental caries?
Feb 2002	Can dental facelifts make you look younger?

Figure 14 Dentistry in the News from the National Library for Health

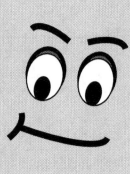

Smile!

Until recently, we had an electronic library for health, or "Nellie" as she was known from her initials NeLH. The National Library for Health is little different, but we have lost the "e-" bit".

This perhaps represents the fact that NeLH has become accepted as part of the infrastructure - Or perhaps merely that it aspires to do so (see earlier comments re changing names!)

Informatics can help you present information

There are a number of situations where you may need to present information to colleagues or patients. The commonest method of presenting information is to use PowerPoint. This is a relatively simple tool to use, and many people feel comfortable using it. However, there are some simple rules that are worth following if you want to communicate effectively:

Ten rules to follow when using PowerPoint

1. Never put more than five points on one slide
2. Keep each point short, use no more than 6 words per point
3. Don't have too many slides, not more than 1 slide per 2 minutes talking
4. Don't use more than two fonts, and don't mix serif and san serif fonts
5. Do not use all the same case, as it's easier to read a mixture of upper and lower case
6. Keep diagrams simple
7. Avoid bright colours
8. Avoid whizzy transitions: they quickly irritate
9. Always check the slide show in situ if you can
10. The talk should drive the slides – not the other way around

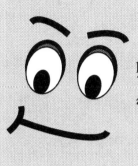

Smile!

And do I follow the rules? Mostly, but I'm not really a rules person, and to prove it I've written a whole book about it. Try *The art of presentation,* to be published by Radcliffe Publishing about the same time as this book.

Visit http://www.radcliffe-oxford.com to find out more

Shameless plug over....

Informatics can help you record your professional development

These days, continuing professional development is a requirement for all staff:

There are a number of electronic resources developed to help you record and structure your professional development activity.

Typically, these will allow you to build up an electronic record of your professional development activity as you go along, enabling you to simply press a button at re-validation time to submit your claim. The best tools will help you structure your practice and reflect upon it:

You may find other useful resources online, for example from your professional association.

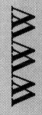

Web link

There are links provided to many of the professional dental associations on the web site accompanying this book. Go to the sections on continuing education to find out more about what's available in your country, state of province.

So you can access information and new knowledge using the technology, and also record your professional development using the technology. Unfortunately, or perhaps fortunately, there's a bit in the middle you have to do yourself, which involves treating patients and thinking through the implications!

RESOLVE NOW TO TRY ADA CE ONLINE

Since its July launch, general dentists, specialists, dental hygienists, assistants, dental students, dental laboratory technicians, administrative personnel, treatment coordinators and dental team members are earning continuing education credits 24 hours each day, seven days a week, 365 days a year at www.ada.org/goto/ceonline.

The cost is $28 per credit hour for members and $42 per credit hour for non-members. Newly reduced pricing for dental team members is $15 per credit hour.

"For me, it's a win-win all the way around," Dr. Schock told ADA News. "ADA CE Online is easy to use, very convenient."

Registrants have access to a course for one year from the date of purchase and can bookmark courses to return to and complete at a later time. Features include a link allowing users to check with their licensing states regarding exact requirements for continuing education. Students receive an electronic letter of completion showing the hour(s) of CE earned.

Compatible for PC and/or Mac users with the connection speed of a dial-up modem (56 kilobits), ADA CE Online also offers toll-free technical support: 1-877-4ADACE1 (1-877-423-2231).

The ADA is a CERP-recognized provider.

Go to ADA CE Online Now! ▶

ADA Quick Links

- Dental Admission Test (DAT)
- National Board Dental Exam (NBDE) Part I
- National Board Dental Exam (NBDE) Part II
- National Board Dental Hygiene Exam (NBDHE)
- ADA CE Online NEW!
- ADA CELL Seminar Series
- Continuing Education Course Listing
- New Dentist News
- Search for Dental Schools and Programs
- A Guide for Developing an Accredited Dental Hygiene Education Program
- Dental Students FAQ
- ADA Annual Session
- Join/Renew Your ADA Membership

Other Sites

- American Student Dental Association
- American Dental Education Association
- Association of Specialized and Professional Accreditation (ASPA)

Figure 15 Education Resources from professional associations, accessible online

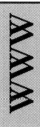

Web link

There are links provided to all of these tools you need on the web site accompanying this book.

☑ Exercise 10

Consider the topic of dental informatics. Identify the first three resources found by five different search engines or databases:

1.   Google.com

2.   Google.co.uk (or other national site if appropriate, eg Google.ca)

3.   Dogpile.com

4.   Google Scholar

5.   Pubmed

Indicate the URL (web address) and whether they are abstracts full resources or restricted access in the "Type" column

Google.com

	Resource identified	Web address (URL)	Type
1			
2			
3			

Google.co.uk etc.

	Resource identified	Web address (URL)	Type
1			
2			
3			

Dogpile

	Resource identified	Web address (URL)	Type
1			
2			
3			

Google Scholar

	Resource identified	Web address (URL)	Type
1			
2			
3			

PubMed

	Resource identified	Web address (URL)	Type
1			
2			
3			

Think Box

Before we leave this chapter, think about the following question:

What are your personal development needs at this time? Can you use these tools to help you find useful information or information about courses or events?

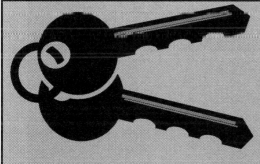

Key points from this chapter

There are a number of areas where the technology can help YOU. In this chapter, I have illustrated how technology can help you:

• Find information

• Present information

• Record your personal development

Chapter 9 Some things that might just make it all worthwhile for your patients

The patients: remember them?

Most dentists are not in it for the money: they do the job because they care about their patients. We have already seen how information technology can prevent harm to patients and improve their care, especially in the area of health promotion. However, we can go further and use information technology to actually give more responsibility for their own care and decisions. We shall consider two key areas:

- Facilitating self management
- Informing patient decisions about treatment

In both cases, the aim is to make sure that patients are properly informed to make the best decisions and give informed consent to treatment.

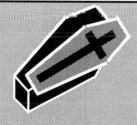

Zombie warning

Many clinicians seem to cling to the idea that patients are incapable of making decisions about their own health.

Some may argue that current trends in obesity provide evidence for this zombie: studies on the lifestyles of health care professionals suggest that the general public may be no worse than clinicians in this regard.

In the UK, the Government commissioned an economist (Derek Wanless) to write two reports on the future viability of public health care [12],[13].

---

[12] *Wanless, D Securing Our Future Health: Taking a Long-Term View, Report for HM Treasury, April 2002, HMSO, London.*

[13] *Wanless D Securing Good Health for the Whole Population, Report for HM Treasury, February 2004, HMSO, London.*

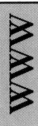

Web link

There are links provided to these reports on the web site accompanying this book.

The reports concluded that the future viability depended upon:

- Greater use of IT to promote smarter working

- Patients taking more responsibility for their own care

This is not rocket science. They are perhaps the greatest universal self evident truths since the American Constitution. However, this has not always been a comfortable message for health care professionals, although dentists as a group have a long tradition of highlighting preventative measures.

The changing role of the clinician

A couple of years ago I was asked to develop an electronic resource to teach people how to find and evaluate health resources on the Internet. The project was funded from resources aimed at patients. However, many of the clinicians felt that it was too dangerous to give such resources directly to patients and the final resources were mediated through clinicians who controlled access to the resources.

A couple of years later, an enhanced resource was developed for ADITUS, the NorthWest of England NHS Library service, and placed on the public portal.

As with many areas, the clinicians role has changed over the years from being an expert and unchallengeable authority to one whose job is now to guide the patient to the best informed decision. Part of this is the ability to advise patients where to look for resources and how to judge whether they are likely to prove reliable.

Table 42 The changing role of the clinician

Many media organisations have invested in online health resources. Generally reliable information may be found in websites run by major media organisations, eg CNN, BBC and the major quality newspapers

Sample patient information from the BBC

Tooth decay: Dr Trisha Macnair

The most common - and most preventable - problem affecting children's teeth is dental decay or caries.

What is it?

Dental decay is a breakdown of the normal hard tissues on the outer surface of the teeth to form a soft cavity or hole. In severe decay, the cavity may be very deep, affecting the nerve and blood vessels in the central pulp.

What causes it?

Bacteria that thrive on the teeth cause tooth decay, particularly when there's a large amount of sugary food debris left in the mouth. The bacteria grow in a sticky coating on the teeth called plaque. They break down food sugars into acids that etch away at the surface enamel, leaking out the calcium and phosphate minerals to soften and destroy the enamel and dentine below.

Frequent sugary foods and drink increases the risk of decay, especially if allowed to bathe the teeth for long periods (for example, if teeth aren't regularly brushed or if a baby sucks on a bottle full of sweet drink).

Who's affected?

Dental decay is very common. The addition of fluoride to toothpaste has helped to protect teeth and cut decay but the continual trend to sweeter snack foods in children's diets is working against this.

At first, tooth decay may not cause any obvious symptoms, especially in milk teeth. But as it progresses it may cause toothache, or sensitivity to hot or cold, or to very sweet foods. If the nerve becomes affected, infection may establish and lead to an abscess, with severe pain, swelling of the jaw and fever.

How's it diagnosed and treated?

Children should have regular check-ups at the dentist (every six months) so that decay can be spotted early. If your child has toothache, always get the advice of a dentist. The dentist will be able to spot decay by examining the teeth and sometimes taking an x-ray to investigate the extent of damage.

Very minor decay can sometimes re-mineralise on its own, if the plaque on the tooth is cleared and better oral hygiene started, with the use of a fluoride gel. But usually a filling will be needed to repair the cavity. If the nerve inside the tooth is infected or damaged the roots of the tooth may need to be filled using a special technique, or the tooth itself removed if it's a baby (milk) tooth.

Prevention is vital to avoid tooth decay

Prevention is vital to avoid tooth decay. Cut down the amount of sweet snacks your child is allowed (including acidic fizzy drinks). Help your children brush their teeth twice a day and after meals, and take them for regular check-ups at the dentist. Make sure that your water supply is fluorinated or discuss fluoride drops with the dentist. You may also want to consider fissure sealant treatment for permanent teeth.

This article was last medically reviewed by Dr Rob Hicks in December 2005.

Figure 16 Information from the Health section of the BBC website

Think Box

Think about the following question:

How do you feel about this information? Would you be happy to recommend it to your patients?

This is often a better way for patients to be guided than simply to type their disease name into Google. Other useful resources to which patients may be pointed are sites like patient UK, which provide details of support groups and patient information leaflets.

In the UK, NHS sites such as the "Dentistry in the News" section of the National Library for Health or NHSDirect Online provide reliable destinations to encourage your patients to visit.

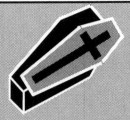

Zombie warning

Faced with the printout wielding patient, some dentists seem to take the view that the Internet is the spawn of the Devil.

The Internet is in reality a vehicle by which patients can access information, some good, some terrible. A better strategy may be to offer more reliable Internet sites for the patient to visit: many patients will be intending to return to the Internet again, so guidance like this may prevent a return visit to a rogue or inappropriate site.

PEDIATRIC SEDATION GUIDELINES ANNOUNCED	A-Z topics
The American Academy of Pediatrics (AAP) and the American Academy of Pediatric Dentistry (AAPD) announced December 4 joint guidelines for all medical and dental practitioners regarding the monitoring and management of pediatric patients during and after sedation. The guidelines recommend: • No administration of sedating medications without the safety net of medical supervision • Careful presedation evaluation for underlying medical or surgical conditions that would place the child at increased risk from sedating medications • Appropriate fasting for elective procedures and a balance between depth of sedation and risk for those who are unable to fast because of the urgent nature of the procedure • A clear understanding of the pharmacokinetic and pharmacodynamic effects of the medications used for sedation as well as an appreciation for drug interactions • Appropriate training and skills in airway management to allow rescue of the patient should there be an adverse response • Age- and size-appropriate equipment for airway management and venous access, appropriate medications and reversal agents • Sufficient numbers of staff to both carry out the procedure and monitor the patient during and after the procedure • Appropriate physiologic monitoring during and after the procedure • A properly equipped and staffed recovery area, recovery to presedation level of consciousness before discharge from medical supervision, and appropriate discharge instructions Access the Complete Guidelines > A-Z Topic: Anesthesia > **Children, Dental Treatment and Anesthesia** When a child needs a difficult or complex dental procedure, the dentist may recommend options for sedation—medications that help control the child's pain or anxiety. Here are questions parents can ask their child's dentist about sedation procedures: • What type of medication(s) will be used and how will they be administered? • What are the possible side effects?	• Bad Breath (Halitosis) • Cleaning Your Teeth and Gums (Oral Hygiene) • Dental Filling Options • Dental Grills (Grillz/Fronts): Video Added • Fluoride & Fluoridation • Meth Mouth: Video Added • Mouth Sores • Oral-Systemic Health sponsored by the makers of Listerine • Osteonecrosis of the Jaw • Periodontal Diseases (Gum Disease) • Root Canal • Tooth Whitening • Wisdom Teeth • X-rays FAQ • And more... **In The News** FDA Safety Alerts (Updated 06/19/06) ADA Offers Tips for Enjoying Holiday Sweets and Keeping that "Sweet Tooth" Intact (Posted 11/17/06)

Figure 17 Patient Information from the American Dental Association.

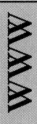

Web link

There are links provided to the patient information resources mentioned here on the web site accompanying this book.

Increasingly such resources are moving away from the static page to full multimedia with animations and full video available to patients as internet bandwidth increases.

The more interactive and impressive such resources become, the greater the risk of misinformation or messages from vested interests being accepted by patients. It is no longer possible for dentist to ignore such initiatives. The role of the dentist is to help patients judge both the effectiveness of any advice offered and its appropriateness for a specific patient. They may choose to refer the patients to resources provided by a professional association.

Within the UK, the NHS has invested heavily in online resources under the NHSDirect banner. However, it is not possible to restrict patients to endorsed sites.

Dental care for babies and children

Print whole article

Send to a friend

Article sections

1. **Introduction**
2. Treatment
3. Prevention
4. Why is it necessary?
5. What to do
6. Selected links

Introduction

Babies start to develop teeth before they are born. The first teeth (also known as milk teeth or deciduous teeth) normally start to break through the gum from at around six to nine months old. Most children will have around eight teeth by their first birthday, although this is just an average. The complete set of twenty milk teeth is usually through by 2 and a half years.

Milk teeth start to fall out when the permanent, adult teeth start to break through the gum. This usually begins around the age of 6 or 7, but continues for several years. Wisdom teeth, or second molars, usually appear between the ages of 17 and 21, but can be much later.

Even small babies are exposed to sugar - the natural sugars in breast milk - which can cause tooth decay, so it is important to start looking after your children's teeth as soon as they appear.

Continue to the next section "Treatment"

Last updated on 02 February 2006 09:52:54

Figure 18 The NHS Direct Online web site

There are many sites with useful information . For example, the Patient UK web site.

Preventing Caries in Children

What is caries?

Caries (tooth decay) is perhaps the most common disease of children in the UK. It is caused by bacteria which act on certain foods in the mouth. Sugary foods and drinks are the worst. The combination of bacteria and food causes acids to form which can slowly dissolve the teeth. If this happens, a filling may be needed. If it is left untreated, the tooth may decay further and need to be removed.

How can caries be prevented?

Brushing teeth

Encourage children to brush their teeth at least twice a day. Start as soon as the first tooth develops in infancy so that you and your child get into a habit. Many children don't like their teeth being brushed at first. However, it is possible to make it into a game when first started. Do persist as it is very important to develop this habit.

By the age of 3 or 4 children can often clean their own teeth (under supervision). A fluoride toothpaste is recommended.

Foods

As far as possible, limit sugary foods and drinks between meals. If you children have sweets, it may be better to eat them all at once as a snack rather than spread them over several hours. Try fruit or raw vegetables as snacks instead. If you child needs medicine, sugar-free medicines are best if they are available.

Fluoride

Fluoride is a chemical that is found naturally in water in very low concentrations. It helps to protect teeth against caries. Some areas have fluoride added to the water supply. This has greatly reduced tooth decay in those areas. It is worth finding out if your area is a fluoride area (your dentist will know). If not, your dentist may advise fluoride drops.

Dental checks

It is worth getting your child used to dental check-ups from an early age. A check up every 6-12 months is best. In some areas, particularly where there is no fluoride in the water supply, a 'sealant' can be placed in the crevices at the back of the teeth by a dentist. This helps protect the teeth from caries and tooth decay. It is 6-7 year olds who may benefit most. A dentist will advise about this.

© EMIS and PIP 2004   Updated: October 2002   CHIQ Accredited

Figure 19 Patient leaflet from the Patient UK web site

More importantly, this will not equip your patients to evaluate web sites for themselves.Here are my checklists for evaluating patient information websites:

Five reasons not to trust a patient information website

1. It is trying to sell something

2. It contains out of date information

3. Links from the site are broken

4. The author/owner is not easily identified

5. The author/owner's credentials are unclear.

Table 43 Five reasons not to trust a patient information website

Additionally, some the advice from perfectly good websites may not be appropriate for your patients

This may be because:

Five reasons why a patient information website may not be appropriate for your patients

1. It recommends treatments not available in your system

2. Your patient has a specific condition which would adversely affect the effectiveness of the treatment

3. Your patient has a specific condition which the treatment would make worse

4. Your patient is too old

5. Your patient is too young

Table 44 Five reasons why a patient information website may not be appropriate for your patients

☑ Exercise 11

Use the Internet search tools from the last chapter to identify five patient information web sites appropriate to your patients

Indicate the URL (web address) and the type of information provided.

	Resource identified	Web address (URL)	Information provided
1			
2			
3			
4			
5			

Think Box

Before we leave this chapter, think about the following question:

How do you judge the quality of information on the Internet?

Do you feel confident advising patients about the quality of information on the Internet?

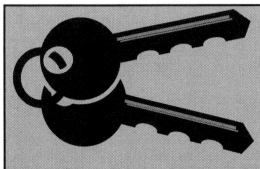

Key points from this chapter

IT can be used to provide patients with information to help them make informed decisions, either in choosing between treatments or through encouraging them to take more responsibility for their own oral health.

In view of the variable quality of information found on the Internet, there is a role for dentists to act as information brokers, to help patients judge the quality of information provided.

Chapter 10 How well do you use information? Here's a model to help you find out

In order to find out how well you use information you need a model with which you can compare your self. We will start by defining three types of information activity.

Activity type	What it's about
Information Technology	The technology associated with information: computers, wires, keyboards, etc. Contrary to popular opinion, whilst technology can really get in the way if it's not right, it cannot deliver benefits on its own
Information Governance	The processes need to ensure that you process information safely, securely and in accordance with best ethical and professional practice.
Information Management	The way you manage your information is crucial to gaining benefits from information. It is all about making sure that you have the right information in the right format at the right time and in the right place

Table 45 Three types of information activity

Each of these elements must be kept in balance with the others:

Activity type	If emphasised at expense of others	If neglected compared to others
Information Technology	The benefits will not be realised from the technology: at best, it will just be under-used and a waste of money: at worst, it may lead to chaos	The lack of appropriate technology can become a major barrier to improvements in practice and information quality
Information Governance	Overzealous governance processes can stifle innovation, and in extremis make the information systems almost impossible to use through too many barriers placed in the way of users.	Inadequate governance procedures can lead to breaches in privacy, consent, inappropriate access. This may result in litigation, bad publicity and professional misconduct proceedings
Information Management	There is little wrong with emphasising information management except where this leads to neglect of information technology and governance processes	If you neglect information management, you will lose many of the potential benefits, waste money on technology and time on establishing governance processes

Table 46 The need to balance activity

For these reasons, we shall build our model in terms of these three strands of activity.

Within each strand we shall use a maturity model approach to model development.

The maturity model approach

The maturity model approach was developed originally by the Software Engineering Institute of the Carnegie-Mellon University for the United States Department of Defense (Watts Humphrys, 1989) [14]. Over the years, I have deployed change management models based upon this approach in medicine, nursing, human resources and information technology and management, and refined the approach.

Five reasons to deploy an approach based upon a maturity model

1. It is a tried and tested approach
2. It recognises that organisations develop at different speeds
3. It can be deployed using straightforward on-line tools
4. It provides information both on current development and what to do next
5. It can be linked to training needs analysis and interventions

Table 47 Five reasons to deploy an approach based upon a maturity model

For our purposes, I shall define specific maturity model known as the Dental Practice Information Maturity Model (DPIMM). Within this approach, the level of organisational capability is defined in terms of one of five levels of maturity:

[14] Humphrey, W.S. (1987) Characterising the software process: a maturity framework. Software Engineering Institute, CMU/SEI-87-TR-11, DTIC Number ADA182895.

Maturity level	Characteristics of this level
Initial	Processes, procedures at this stage are ad hoc. The practice will have a computer system, but it is used by the enthusiasts amongst the dentists, and for mandated activities, or those with an immediat payback, eg billing; governance aspects are covered by individual profesisonal codes of practice, and information management is neglected
Improving	The practice has started to define its processes. The dentists have started to use the information system for clinical purposes. Basic policies are defined for consent and confidentiality. Thought has been given to the information to be collected and used within the practice
Systematic	The practice has a full set of policies and processes. Information technology is used throughouit the practice. Comprehensive governance policies are in place to protect privacy. Basic indicators are used to monitor performance in respect of the use of information.
Payback	The practice uses information across most of its activity. Informtaion is generated routinely in support of audit and performance management. Activities for health promotion are routinely supported by automated protocols, and data is input using protocols to help standardise data entry. Communications with the wider health community and other agencies are handle electronically. Data is recorded to externally agreed standards.
Optimising	Information is embedded within the culture of the practice. The practice operates in a paperless fashion both internally and externally. Information is used to review dental and business practices to underpin a culture of continuous improvement.

Table 48 Maturity levels for the Dental Practice Information Maturity Model

In order to balance information technology, information governance and information maturity activities, the DPIMM model defines a distinct maturity for each strand. In an ideal world, the maturity level for each would be the same indicating balanced development. Certainly, variations in maturity should not exceed one level between the strands.

To evaluate your information maturity, start by considering your information technology maturity using the electronic questionnaire.

The Dental Practice Information Maturity Model

Select an information domain to audit. or click here to find out more, by going to IT4Dentists.com

The maturity model is divided into three domains. Select a domain for your maturity audit or your training needs analysis:

— Information Technology maturity audit

— Information Management maturity audit

— Information Governance maturity audit

— Information Technology training needs audit

— Information Management training needs audit

— Information Governance training needs audit

Click here for an explanation of the proficiency scale used in the training needs analysis

(c) Professor Alan Gillies, 2006.

Figure 20 The opening screen for the Dental Practice Information Maturity Model on-line tools

Select the first option, labelled Information Technology maturity audit. This stream of the model is concerned with the technology, but also with the management processes rquired to manage the risks associated with the technology, as described in Chapter 7

At this stage, the questionnaire asks only two questions about the technology itself, with the rest concerned with management processes associated with the introduction of the technology.

Moving the mouse over the questions highlights explanatory text about the question: moving the mouse the mouse over the warning triangle highlights the risks of inaction in respect of this item.

In the event of a problem, without a backup, you may suffer serious data loss

Figure 21 Stage 1 screen of the information technology maturity audit: warning of inaction

If you have this level of technology available, then tick the option box and then select the "Analyse Results" button. Move through the remainder of the questions, ticking those options that you can answer "yes".

Information Technology Stage 1: Initial

Click the tick box where you can answer "yes" to the following questions.

1.1 Do you have a computer system in the practice?

1.2 Do all of the dentists in the practice have access to a computer system in the place where they deliver care?

1.3 Do you have a log of problems and errors with the systems?

1.4 Does the organisation use adequate virus protection software?

1.5 Do you back up all your data at least once a week?

1.6 Do you back up new information every day?

1.7 Is the system protected against an interruption in the power supply?

Click the Analyse button when you have completed this page. Analyse results (c) Professor Alan Gillies, 2006.

Figure 22 Stage 1 screen of the information technology maturity audit

If you can answer all the items on this page, you will see the confirmatory dialog box to show that you have achieved this level of maturity. Select OK to accept and progress to the next level.

[Javascript Application]

Your responses indicate that you have met all the requirements of this level.

Click on OK to proceed to the next level or Cancel to quit

| OK | Cancel |

Figure 23 Confirmatory dialog box when level is complete.

Click OK to accept. This takes you to level 2.

Information Technology Stage 2: Improving

Click the tick box where you can answer "yes" to the following questions.

2.1 Are all the surgery sites linked through a common computer system capable of running the same electronic dental records system?

2.2 Do all practice surgeries have access to Internet and Email facilities?

2.3 Is there a regular schedule of electrical safety inspections for the IT system?

2.4 Is there a regular schedule of inspections of security systems?

2.5 Does the organisation have a policy to prevent viruses entering the system where possible, through limits on access of floppy disks and or Email to the system?

2.6 Has a system been set up to monitor, investigate and system errors?

2.7 Has an audit been carried out to establish current levels of user knowledge regarding the system ?

2.8 Do you remove a copy of all your data to a safe remote location at least once a month?

Click the Analyse button when you have completed this page. Analyse results (c) Professor Alan Gillies, 2006.

Figure 24 DPIMM IT Stage 2 audit items

At this stage of the information technology stream of the DPIMM, there are once again only two questions that directly relate to implementation of technology and the remainder relate to its management:

Are all the surgery sites linked through a common computer system capable of running the same electronic dental records system?

Do all practice surgeries have access to Internet and Email facilities?

The remainder of the questions relate to the management of the technology. If you are able to answer all these questions positively, then repeat the process to move to level 3. Level 3 of the information technology audit involves more questions about technological facilities as well as processes.

Information Technology Stage 3: Systematic

Click the tick box where you can answer "yes" to the following questions.

3.1 Does the practice have a central server to provide a common repository for electronic patient records?

3.2 Are all the dentist computer systems using the same application?

3.3 Are all the dentist computer systems using the same software version?

3.4 Does the system allow for information to be pulled into the electronic record directly from laboratory results?

3.5 Do you have secure messaging system to transmit and receive secure messages to local hospitals and other health care facilities?

3.6 Are the individual dentist systems connected to a common practice server?

3.7 Are the individual dentist systems synchronised in near real time to a common practice server?

3.8 Have the individual dentist systems been harmonised to remove duplicate records?

3.9 Does the computer system provide connectivity to a suitable web portal and other resources for Continuing Medical Education?

3.10 Does the computer system provide connectivity to allow secure transmission of electronic patient data?

3.11 Does the computer system provide facilities to store images digitally?

3.12 Has a system been set up to automatically report system errors to the supplier?

3.13 Has a system been set up to notify users of problems?

Click the Analyse button when you have completed this page. Analyse results (c) Professor Alan Gillies, 2006.

Figure 25 Stage 3 of the DPIMM Information Techology Maturity Audit

Complete the options that apply to you, then select "Analyse results".

If you do not select all the options as completed, then you will see the report screen.

This indicates your current maturity level and indicates the tasks necessary to move to the next maturity level. You may save or print the report for audit purposes, and the computer will date the form for this purpose. The sample report shown in Table 49 is based upon a nil submssion at level 3, showing all the tasks necessary to move from IT level 2 to level 3.

Your current capability level is Stage 2: Improving

In order to achieve the next level(Stage 3: Systematic)in information technology, you need to

- install a central practice server to provide a common repository for electronic patient records
- install the same dental records application on all dentist computers
- install the same software version on all dentist computers
- set up the system to pull information into the electronic record directly from laboratory results
- establish a secure messaging system to transmit and receive secure messages to local hospitals and other health care facilities
- connect individual dentist systems to a common practice server
- synchronise individual dentist systems to a common practice server in near real time
- harmonise individual dentist systems to remove duplicate records
- connect individual dentist systems to a suitable web portal and other resources for Continuing Education
- provide secure facilities to transmit electronic patient data
- provide secure facilities to store images digitally
- enable remote monitoring of your system
- establish a process to notify users of problems

Press [Ctrl] and P to print this report

Press [Ctrl] and [S] to save this report on your computer. It is recommended that you save the report as a plain text (.txt) file

To keep this audit as a record, print off this page, and sign below:

Signed: _____ **Print Name:** _____

Date of Audit: November 27, 106

(c) Professor Alan Gillies, 2006. All results are dependent upon the data entered. No responsibility can be accepted by the supplier for consequences arising from the results

Table 49 Sample report from the DPIMM IT maturity model

Once you have established your information technology maturity, you should consider your information management maturity. If it emerges lower than your IT maturity then you are not getting the best from your technology. If it emerges higher, then you are doing well, but the technology is likely to become a barrier soon

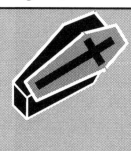

Zombie warning

The view that Information Technology is a "magic bullet" solution, and can solve all your problems, is remarkably persistent in the face of so many IT systems in health care applications failing to deliver real benefits through a failure to appreciate the information management implications.

Consider the following information management audit, for a dental practice with level 2 information management maturity, but no level 3 activity.

Information Management Stage 1: Initial

Click the tick box where you can answer "yes" to the following questions.

1.1 Do you have a signed commitment from all contributing dentists to share data and to implement common data standards across the practice?

1.2 Do you use an IT system for administration?

1.3 Do you have a patient registry where each patient is uniquely identifiable by a unique identifier?

Click the Analyse button when you have completed this page. Analyse results (c) Professor Alan Gillies, 2006.

Figure 26 Stage 1 audit items of the DPIMM Information Management Maturity Audit

Information Management Stage 2: Improving

Click the tick box where you can answer "yes" to the following questions.

2.1 Do you use a IT system for any clinical functions?

2.2 Do you use a IT system to record activities for billing?

2.3 Do you have a patient registry which can identify groups by age and sex?

2.4 Do all the health care professionals within the practice use the electronic patient record to find information about patients?

2.5 Do you use a IT system to check your prescribing for errors?

2.6 Do you record drug allergies in your patient registry?

2.7 Do you use a IT system to issue prescriptions?

2.8 Do you carry out a regular audit of the quality of your data?

Click the Analyse button when you have completed this page. Analyse results (c) Professor Alan Gillies, 2006.

Figure 27 Stage 2 Screen of DPIMM Information Management Maturity Audit

If you do not tick any othe items at this stage you will see a complete list of the actions required to achieve level 3 maturity for information management maturity.

The final maturity audit is for information governance. As the use of information incresaes in both activity and complexity, so the governnace issues increase. It is important to balance maturity in information management and technology with appropriate governance activity to keep patient data safe and prevent inappropriate release of data.

This is not simply dental data: there are recorded cases of where information released in good faith about attendance for a routine appointment to a partner led to a significant complaint from a patient.

The maturity model for information governance is organised into five maturity levels mirroring the levels of the other streams.

Select the Information Governance maturity model from the opening screen to carry out an audit.

Information Management Stage 3: Systematic

Click the tick box where you can answer "yes" to the following questions.

3.1 Does every member of the practice have access to the IT system ?

3.2 Do all the dentists within the practice record their care within the electronic patient record?

3.3 Do you record key dental data on your IT system according to standards agreed across your practice?

3.4 Do you use an IT system to check prescriptions for contraindications and allergies?

3.5 Do you use an IT system to issue all prescriptions?

3.6 Do you access laboratory results electronically?

3.7 Do you request laboratory tests electronically?

3.8 Do you store X-rays digitally?

3.9 Do you use your IT system for monitoring smoking status?

3.10 Do you use your IT system for routine recalls of patients for periodic check-ups?

3.11 Do you use your IT system to send out automated reminders by email and/or SMS texts?

3.12 Do you use your IT system to identify and monitor specific groups of patients?

3.13 Do you use secure email for transmission of messages?

3.14 Do you transmit prescriptions to pharmacies electronically?

3.15 Do you access remote information and educational material using your IT facilities?

3.16 Do you access knowledge resources for care and continuing medical education electronically?

Click the Analyse button when you have completed this page. Analyse results (c) Professor Alan Gillies, 2006.

Figure 28 Stage 3 Screen of DPIMM Information Management Maturity Audit

Your current capability level is Stage 2: Improving

In order to achieve the next level(Stage 3: Systematic) in information management, you need to:

- ensure that every member of the practice has access to the IT system

- ensure that all the dentists within the practice record their care within the electronic patient record

- record key dental data on your IT system according to standards agreed across your practice

- use an IT system to check prescriptions for contraindications and allergies

- use an IT system to issue all prescriptions

- access laboratory results electronically

- request laboratory tests electronically

- store X-rays digitally

- use your IT system for monitoring smoking status

- use your IT system for routine recalls of patients for periodic check-ups

- use your IT system to send out automated reminders by email and/or SMS texts

- use your IT system to identify and monitor specific groups of patients

- use secure email for transmission of messages

- transmit your prescriptions to pharmacies electronically

- access remote information and educational material using your IT facilities

- access knowledge resources for care and continuing medical education electronically

Press [Ctrl] and P to print this report

Press [Ctrl] and [S] to save this report on your computer. It is recommended that you save the report as a plain text (.txt) file

To keep this audit as a record, print off this page, and sign below:

Signed: _____ **Print Name:** _____

Date of Audit: November 28, 2006

(c) Professor Alan Gillies, 2006. All results are dependent upon the data entered. No responsibility can be accepted by the supplier for consequences arising from the results

Table 50 Sample report from DPIMM IM maturity model

Information Governance Stage 1: Initial

Click the tick box where you can answer "yes" to the following questions.

1.1 Is there any training provision for knowledgeable consent?

1.2 Are standard consent forms available?

1.3 Has awareness training for staff been established in determining specific needs of patients in the establishment of knowledgeable consent?

1.4 Has awareness training for staff been established in the implications of the relevant disability discrimination legislation in the establishment of knowledgeable consent?

1.5 Has awareness training for staff been established in determining specific needs of children in the establishment of knowledgeable consent?

1.6 Has awareness training for staff been established in determining specific needs of minority patients in the establishment of knowledgeable consent?

1.7 Has awareness training for staff been established in the implications of relevant racial discrimination legislation in the establishment of knowledgeable consent?

1.8 Is information provided for patients on the proposed uses of information about them?

1.9 Has a staff code of conduct in respect of privacy been written?

1.10 Are basic privacy & security requirements included in some staff induction procedures?

1.11 Is there any training provision for privacy?

1.12 Are privacy requirements included in contracts for some staff ?

1.13 Are basic agreements of undertaking signed by relevant support organisations and contractors, and by all others with access to personal data?

1.14 Is there any training provision for information security?

1.15 Is there any training provision for information sharing?

1.16 Is ownership established for some information or data sets?

1.17 Has an awareness programme for personal responsibilities for information security been carried out?

1.18 Has an awareness programme for organisational responsibilities for information security carried out?

1.19 Are there any information security incident control or investigation procedures established?

1.20 Are there basic reporting procedures for major incidents or problem areas?

1.21 Are systems users encouraged to change passwords regularly?

1.22 Are there any access controls established?

1.23 Are there any lockable rooms and/or cabinets available?

Click the Analyse button when you have completed this page. Analyse results (c) Professor Alan Gillies, 2006.

Figure 29 Stage 1 Screen of DPIMM Information Governance Maturity Audit

Information Governance Stage 2: Improving

Click the tick box where you can answer "yes" to the following questions.

2.1 Is training available for all staff in knowledgeable consent?

2.2 Are standard consent forms are in use throughout organisation?

2.3 Are procedures established for determining specific needs of patients in the establishment of knowledgeable consent?

2.4 Are procedures established for determining specific needs of children in the establishment of knowledgeable consent?

2.5 Are procedures established for determining specific needs of minority patients in the establishment of knowledgeable consent that meet the requirements of relevant racial discrimination legislation ?

2.6 Is there an active information campaign established to promote patient awareness of the proposed uses of information about them?

2.7 Are basic privacy & security requirements included in all staff induction Procedures?

2.8 Is training available for all staff in privacy?

2.9 Have the principal information flows containing personally identifiable information been identified and comprehensively mapped?

2.10 Has a register of ownership established for some information or data sets?

2.11 Are any locally agreed protocols established governing the sharing of personally identifiable information with other directorates and organisations?

2.12 Is training available for all staff in information security?

2.13 Is training available for all staff in information sharing?

 2.14 Is there a Security Policy available?

2.15 Are the personal responsibilities for information security documented?

2.16 Are the organisational responsibilities for information security documented?

2.17 Is a risk management programme underway and reports available?

2.18 Are the procedures for information security incident control documented and accessible to staff to ensure incidents are reported and investigated promptly? 2.19 Are there processes established to ensure security is monitored and lessons are learnt from security incidents?

2.20 Are password changes enforced on a regular basis?

2.21 Is there an initial assessment of staff training needs?

Click the Analyse button when you have completed this page. Analyse results (c) Professor Alan Gillies, 2006.

Figure 30 Stage 2 Screen of DPIMM Information Governance Maturity Audit

Information Governance Stage 3: Systematic

Click the tick box where you can answer "yes" to the following questions.

3.1. Are standard procedures for establishing consent established throughout the practice?

3.2. Are standard procedures for verifying consent established throughout the practice?

3.3. Are procedures in use across organisation for determining specific needs of patients in the establishment of knowledgeable consent?

3.4. Are procedures in use across organisation for determining specific needs of children in the establishment of knowledgeable consent?

3.5. Are procedures in use across organisation for determining specific needs of minority patients in the establishment of knowledgeable consent that meet the requirements of relevant racial discrimination legislation ?

3.6. Is there an active information campaign supported by comprehensive arrangements for patients with special/different needs?

3.7. Are agreed protocols established to govern the sharing and use of all confidential information?

3.8. Do formal contractual arrangements exist with all contractors and support organisations?

3.9. Have all information flows containing personally identifiable information been identified and comprehensively mapped?

3.10. Is ownership established and registered for all information or datasets?

3.11. Have justifying purposes and staff access restrictions been agreed by the practice?

3.12. Have all partner organisations been clearly identified and information requirements understood and documented?

3.13. Is the Security Policy reviewed annually and reissued as appropriate?

3.14. Is the responsibility for information security coordinated at a high level by one or more individuals in the practice?

3.15. Does a formal programme for information security exist with regular reviews, outcome reports and recommendations provided for senior management?

3.16. Does a dissemination mechanism exist to share findings of risk management programme with relevant staff?

3.17. Is a dissemination mechanism established to ensure that the practice share with staff the implications of all identified information security incidents?

3.18. Has the staff code of conduct in respect of privacy has been agreed by relevant staff organisations?

3.19. Has the staff code of conduct in respect of privacy has been circulated to all staff (including switchboard and post room staff)?

3.20. Has a comprehensive awareness raising exercise been undertaken around privacy & security requirements?

3.21. Has there been a systematic evaluation of training that has occurred as part of supervision and appraisal process?

3.22. Are privacy requirements included in all staff contracts?

Click the Analyse button when you have completed this page. Analyse results (c) Professor Alan Gillies, 2006.

Figure 31 Stage 3 Screen of DPIMM Information Governance Maturity Audit

Your current capability level is Stage 2: Improving

In order to achieve the next level(Stage 3: Systematic) in information governance, you need to:

- ensure that standard procedures for establishing consent are in place throughout organisation
- ensure that standard procedures for verifying consent are established throughout organisation
- ensure that procedures are in use across organisation for determining specific needs of patients in the establishment of knowledgeable consent
- ensure that procedures are in use across organisation for determining specific needs of children in the establishment of knowledgeable consent
- ensure that procedures are in use across organisation for determining specific needs of minority patients in the establishment of knowledgeable consent that meet the requirements of relevant racial discrimination legislation
- ensure that there is an active information campaign supported by comprehensive arrangements for patients with special/different needs
- ensure that agreed protocols are established to govern the sharing and use of all confidential information
- ensure that formal contractual arrangements exist with all contractors and support organisations
- ensure that all information flows containing personally identifiable information been identified and comprehensively mapped
- ensure that ownership is established and registered for all information or datasets
- agree justifying purposes and staff access restrictions across the practice
- identify all partner directorates and organisations and understand and document information requirements
- review the Security Policy annually and reissue as appropriate
- co-ordinate responsibility for information security at a high level by one or more individuals
- implement a formal programme for information security with regular reviews, outcome reports and recommendations provided for senior management
- implement a dissemination mechanism exist to share findings of risk management programme with relevant staff
- implement a dissemination mechanism established to ensure that the practice share with staff the implications of all identified information security incidents
- agree the staff code of conduct in respect of privacy with relevant staff organisations
- circulate the staff code of conduct in respect of privacy to all staff (including switchboard and post room staff)
- undertake a comprehensive awareness raising exercise around privacy & security requirements

- carry out a systematic evaluation of training as part of supervision and appraisal process
- ensure that privacy requirements included in all staff contracts

Press [Ctrl] and P to print this report

Press [Ctrl] and [S] to save this report on your computer. It is recommended that you save the report as a plain text (.txt) file

To keep this audit as a record, print off this page, and sign below:

Signed: _____ **Print Name:** _____

Date of Audit: November 28, 2006

Table 51 sample report from DPIMM IG maturity model

If you click Analyse results and you are not able to complete all the items for this level, then you will see the information governance maturity report, such as the one shown in Table 51.

However, an organisation cannot improve unless its staff are competent to carry out their roles. The model measures the proficiency of staff in terms of a model developed from earlier work by the author and a colleague[15]. The model of proficiency is defined for each information competency area in terms of the scale shown in Table 52.

The practitioner can use the supplied tools to record their perceived proficiency in each competency area against that required for that role in a practice of that maturity. This may usefully be done as part of an annual staff review.

As the practice becomes more mature in their use of information, then the staff proficiency levels required to achieve competence increase.

Each member of staff enters their perceived proficiency for each strand of information activity, together with their role and the practice maturity:

[15] *Gillies and Howard (2003) Competency in Health Care, Radcliffe Publishing, Abingdon and Seattle, based upon earlier work by Benner P (1984) Novice to expert*

Level	Description
Level 0	This does not form a part of the current or future role of the worker
Level 1- Foundation	The practitioner would only practice whilst under the direct supervision of others more proficient in this competency. (This level of attainment may apply to the practitioner gaining experience and developing skills and knowledge in the competency)
Level 2- Intermediate	The practitioner can demonstrate acceptable performance in the competency and has coped with enough real situations in the workplace to require less supervision and guidance, but they are not expected to demonstrate full competence or practice autonomously.
Level 3- Proficient	A practitioner who consistently applies the competency standard. The practitioner demonstrates competence through the skills and ability to practice safely and effectively without the need for direct supervision. (The Proficient Practitioner may practice autonomously, and supervise others, within a restricted range of competences.
Level 4- Advanced	The Advanced Practitioner is autonomous and reflexive, perceives situations as wholes, delivers care safely and accurately and is aware of current best practice. Advanced Practitioners understand a situation as a whole because they perceive it's meaning in terms of long-term goals.
Level 5- Expert	The Expert Practitioner is able to demonstrate a deeper understanding of the situation and contributes to the development and dissemination of knowledge through the teaching and development of others. The Expert Practitioner is likely to have their own caseload and provide advice, guidance and leadership to other professionals involved in the delivery or provision of health and social care.

Table 52 Proficiency scale used within DPIMM

Information Technology Training Needs Analysis

Rate your proficiency in each of these areas. Ideally, do this exercise with a manager or colleague

Personal computers & peripheral equipment	Intermediate
Using mobile communications and computing	Intermediate
File management	Intermediate
Using a network	Intermediate
Using word processing software	Intermediate
Using spreadsheet software	Intermediate
Using database software	Intermediate
Using presentations software	Intermediate
Using electronic mail	Intermediate
Using Internet / intranet	Intermediate
Using electronic diaries	Intermediate

Please make sure that you are familiar with the rating scale before attempting this exercise!

Enter the practice Information technology maturity	Improving
Select your role here	Dentist
Enter your name here	Anna Scetic

Click the Analyse button when you have completed this page. Analyse results (c) Professor Alan Gillies, 2006.

Figure 32 Training needs analysis screen for IT

The computer compares the values entered with a table of values like the one below and produces a training needs report.

Required proficiency for dentists in information technology

Competency	Role	DPIMM Maturity level					
Area	Dentists	0	1	2	3	4	5
Personal computers & peripheral equipment		0	2	2	3	3	3
Using mobile communications and computing		0	0	0	1	2	3
File management		0	2	2	3	3	3
Using a network		0	1	2	3	3	3
Using word processing software		0	2	2	3	3	3
Using spreadsheet software		0	1	2	3	3	3
Using database software		0	0	1	2	3	3
Using presentations software		0	1	2	3	3	3
Using electronic mail		0	2	2	3	3	3
Using Internet / intranet		0	2	2	3	3	3

Table 53 Required proficiency values are stored for each role at each maturity level.

Training needs analysis report: A Dentist

From your data entered, and your role, and the maturity of the practice, the model suggests you need training in:

- Personal computers & peripheral equipment

Press [Ctrl] and P to print this report

Press [Ctrl] and [S] to save this report on your computer. It is recommended that you save the report as a plain text (.txt) file

To keep this analysis as a record, print off this page, and sign below:

Signed: _____ : A Dentist

Date of Audit: November 28, 2006

Table 54 Sample IT training needs report for a dentist

The model is defined for four staff roles: Dentists, Nurses, Manager, Admin staff

The process is repeated for the other two strands

Information Technology Training Needs Analysis

Rate your proficiency in each of these areas. Ideally, do this exercise with a manager or colleague

Clinical systems	Intermediate
Non-clinical systems	Intermediate
Data quality	Intermediate
Coding	Intermediate
Identifying information needs	Intermediate
Obtaining information	Intermediate
Analysing and interpreting information	Intermediate
Communicating information	Intermediate
Clinical record keeping	Intermediate
Clinical decision support	Intermediate
Clinical communications	Intermediate
Clinical audit	Intermediate
Evidence-based practice	Intermediate
Local dental information strategy	Intermediate
National dental information strategy	Intermediate

Please make sure that you are familiar with the rating scale before attempting this exercise!

Enter the practice Information technology maturity	Improving
Select your role here	Dentist
Enter your name here	Anna Scetic

Click the Analyse button when you have completed this page. Analyse results (c) Professor Alan Gillies, 2006.

Figure 33 Training needs questionnaire for information management

Information Governance Training Needs Analysis

Rate your proficiency in each of these areas. Ideally, do this exercise with a manager or colleague

Underlying ethical principles	Intermediate
Knowledgeable consent	Intermediate
Consent involving children	Intermediate
Consent involving patients with specific needs	Intermediate
Consent to use of information for research	Intermediate
Consent to participation in experimental procedures	Intermediate
Privacy	Intermediate
Anonymity of data	Intermediate
Patient consent to disclosure	Intermediate
Disclosing information to immediate colleagues	Intermediate
Privacy issues around sharing with other agencies	Intermediate
Good practice in record keeping	Intermediate
Changing needs of confidentiality with electronic records	Intermediate
Privacy issues for multiple purposes	Intermediate
Protecting information against accidental damage	Intermediate
Protecting information against unauthorised access	Intermediate
Protecting information against malicious damage	Intermediate
The implications of local privacy legislation	Intermediate
The implications of national privacy legislation	Intermediate

Please make sure that you are familiar with the rating scale before attempting this exercise!

Enter the practice Information technology maturity	Improving
Select your role here	Dentist
Enter your name here	Anna Scetic

Click the Analyse button when you have completed this page. Analyse results (c) Professor Alan Gillies, 2006.

Figure 34 Training needs questionnaire for information governance

Think Box

Before we leave this chapter think about the following question:

What would the DPIMM tools say about your practice?

In the next chapter, we shall apply the DPIMM tool to a case study practice to see what it can tell us about a practice.

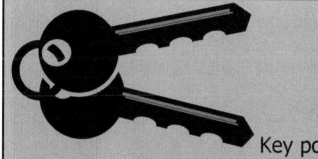

Key points from this chapter

The Dental Practice Information Maturity Model can be used to assess the effectiveness of your use of information.

It is important to keep your information technology, management and governance in balance.

It is important to ensure that staff have the required skills. As your practices matures in its use of information, the skill levels required by staff will increase and change.

Chapter 11 A case study practice evaluated using DPIMM

The following case study is a fictional practice constructed from a number of dental practices with which I am familiar to illustrate the use of the model. The names have been constructed

> Dentown Dental Practice has 5 dentists working at three different locations in a town of approximately 80,000 people, on the edge of a large conurbation. The practice serves a total of 7,500 patients. They operate a private adult practice, with about half their patients belonging to a private dental insurance plan. In addition they offer a public (NHS) children's dental service.
>
> They have a strong relationship with a local orthodontist, and employ 5 dental nurses and a dental hygenist within the practice
>
> The practice has just taken delivery of a shiny new computer system, which allows the use of centralised records for the first time, and information to be shared across the different sites.

Table 55 The case study practice

The practice manager, Penny Counter, has just undertaken a DPIMM audit across the practice to see how the practice is making use of its shiny new IT system.

She is able to complete the opening screen of the IT audit, answering "yes" to all of the following questions:

1.1 Do you have a computer system in the practice?	Yes
1.2 Do all of the dentists in the practice have access to a computer system in the place where they deliver care?	Yes
1.3 Do you have a log of problems and errors with the systems?	Yes
1.4 Does the organisation use adequate virus protection software?	Yes
1.5 Do you back up all your data at least once a week?	Yes
1.6 Do you back up new information every day?	Yes
1.7 Is the system protected against an interruption in the power supply?	Yes

Table 56 Stage 1 IT DPIMM Responses from Dentown Dental Practice

At the next screen she is able to answer "yes" to only the first two items

She selects "Analyse Results" and proceeds to the next screen. However, she is surprised to find that in spite of the shiny new technology, the practice is yet to achieve maturity level 2 (Improving) in Information Technology:

2.1 Are all the surgery sites linked through a common computer system capable of running the same electronic dental records system?	Yes
2.2 Do all practice surgeries have access to Internet and Email facilities?	Yes
2.3 Is there a regular schedule of electrical safety inspections for the IT system?	No
2.4 Is there a regular schedule of inspections of security systems?	No
2.5 Does the organisation have a policy to prevent viruses entering the system where possible, through limits on access of floppy disks and or Email to the system?	No
2.6 Has a system been set up to monitor, investigate and system errors?	No
2.7 Has an audit been carried out to establish current levels of user knowledge regarding the system ?	No
2.8 Do you remove a copy of all your data to a safe remote location at least once a month?	No

Table 57 Stage 2 IT DPIMM Responses from Dentown Dental Practice

Your current capability level is Stage 1: Initial

In order to achieve the next level (Stage 2: Improving)in information technology, you need to:

- establish a regular schedule of electrical safety inspections for the IT system
- establish a regular schedule of inspections of security systems
- implement a policy to prevent viruses entering the system where possible, through limits on access of floppy disks and or Email to the system
- establish a system been set up to monitor, investigate and system errors
- carry out an audit been to establish current levels of user knowledge regarding the system
- remove a copy of all your data to a safe remote location at least once a month

Press [Ctrl] and P to print this report

Press [Ctrl] and [S] to save this report on your computer. It is recommended that you save the report as a plain text (.txt) file

To keep this audit as a record, print off this page, and sign below:

Signed: _____Penny Counter_____ **Print Name** _____ Penny Counter _____

Date of Audit: December 6, 2006

(c) Professor Alan Gillies, 2006. All results are dependent upon the data entered. No responsibility can be accepted by the supplier for consequences arising from the results

Table 58 DPIMM IT report for Dentown Dental Practice

The reason for this low level of maturity is due to the lack of processes to manage the new technology, and the consequent risks to which the system and the practice are exposed.

Penny moved along to information management, and was relieved to be able to complete the opening screen.

1.1 Do you have a signed commitment from all contributing dentists to share data and to implement common data standards across the practice?	Yes
1.2 Do you use an IT system for administration?	Yes
1.3 Do you have a patient registry where each patient is uniquely identifiable by a unique identifier?	Yes

Table 59 Stage 1 IM DPIMM Responses from Dentown Dental Practice

However, she learnt that the practice had yet to achieve level 2 maturity in information management either:

2.1 Do you use a IT system for any clinical functions?	Yes
2.2 Do you use a IT system to record activities for billing?	Yes
2.3 Do you have a patient registry which can identify groups by age and sex?	No
2.4 Do all the health care professionals within the practice use the electronic patient record to find information about patients?	No
2.5 Do you use a IT system to check your prescribing for errors?	No
2.6 Do you record drug allergies in your patient registry?	No
2.7 Do you use a IT system to issue prescriptions?	No
2.8 Do you carry out a regular audit of the quality of your data?	No

Table 60 Stage 2 IM DPIMM Responses from Dentown Dental Practice

The resulting report highlighted the current issues in information management.

Your current capability level is Stage 1: Initial

In order to achieve the next level (Stage 2: Improving) in information management, you need to:

- ensure that all the health care professionals within the practice use the electronic patient record to find information about patients.

- use an IT system to check your prescribing for errors to prevent errors

- use the IT system to record drug allergies in your patient registry.

- use an IT system to issue prescriptions.

- carry out regular audits of the quality of your data.

Press [Ctrl] and P to print this report

Press [Ctrl] and [S] to save this report on your computer. It is recommended that you save the report as a plain text (.txt) file

To keep this audit as a record, print off this page, and sign below:

Signed: _____Penny Counter_____   **Print Name** _____ Penny Counter _____

Date of Audit: December 6, 2006

(c) Professor Alan Gillies, 2006. All results are dependent upon the data entered. No responsibility can be accepted by the supplier for consequences arising from the results

Table 61 DPIMM IM report for Dentown Dental Practice

Finally, Penny audited the practice against the information governance stream. The first screen had items she was not able to complete, and as a result, the practice was not able to achieve information governance maturity level 1 (Initial).

1.1 Is there any training provision for knowledgeable consent?	Yes
1.2 Are standard consent forms available?	Yes
1.3 Has awareness training for staff been established in determining specific needs of patients in the establishment of knowledgeable consent?	No
1.4 Has awareness training for staff been established in the implications of the relevant disability discrimination legislation in the establishment of knowledgeable consent?	No
1.5 Has awareness training for staff been established in determining specific needs of children in the establishment of knowledgeable consent?	No
1.6 Has awareness training for staff been established in determining specific needs of minority patients in the establishment of knowledgeable consent?	No
1.7 Has awareness training for staff been established in the implications of relevant racial discrimination legislation in the establishment of knowledgeable consent?	No
1.8 Is information provided for patients on the proposed uses of information about them?	No
1.9 Has a staff code of conduct in respect of privacy been written?	Yes
1.10 Are basic privacy & security requirements included in some staff induction procedures?	No
1.11 Is there any training provision for privacy?	Yes
1.12 Are privacy requirements included in contracts for some staff?	No
1.13 Are basic agreements of undertaking signed by relevant support organisations and contractors, and by all others with access to personal data?	No
1.14 Is there any training provision for information security?	No
1.15 Is there any training provision for information sharing?	No
1.16 Is ownership established for some information or data sets?	No
1.17 Has an awareness programme for personal responsibilities for information security been carried out?	No
1.18 Has an awareness programme for organisational responsibilities for information security carried out?	No
1.19 Are there any information security incident control or investigation procedures established?	No
1.20 Are there basic reporting procedures for major incidents or problem areas?	No
1.21 Are systems users encouraged to change passwords regularly?	No
1.22 Are there any access controls established?	No
1.23 Are there any lockable rooms and/or cabinets available?	Yes

Table 62 Stage 1 IG DPIMM Responses from Dentown Dental Practice

Your current capability level is not yet measurable!

In order to achieve the next level (Stage1: Initial) in information governance, you need to:

- establish awareness training for staff in determining specific needs of patients in the establishment of knowledgeable consent
- establish awareness training for staff in the implications of the relevant disability discrimination legislation in the establishment of knowledgeable consent
- establish awareness training for staff in determining specific needs of children in the establishment of knowledgeable consent
- establish awareness training for staff in determining specific needs of minority patients in the establishment of knowledgeable consent
- establish awareness training for staff in the implications of relevant racial discrimination legislation in the establishment of knowledgeable consent
- provide information for patients on the proposed uses of information about them
- include basic privacy & security requirements in priority staff induction procedures
- included privacy requirements in contracts for priority staff
- get basic agreements of undertaking signed by relevant support organisations and contractors for service provision, and by other agencies and individuals with access to personal data
- provide training in information security
- provide training in information sharing
- establish ownership for priority information or data sets
- carry out an awareness programme for personal responsibilities for information security
- carry out an awareness programme for organisational responsibilities for information security
- establish information security incident control or investigation procedures in priority areas
- establish basic reporting procedures for major incidents or problem areas
- encourage systems users to change passwords regularly
- establish access controls in high risk areas

Table 63 DPIMM Information governance report for Dentown Dental Practice

Penny Counter calls a practice meeting to discuss the findings from the audit. The dentists are dismayed. They argue that the omissions are in the areas of policies and training for staff. The outcome of the meeting is more work for Penny: she is asked to carry out a training needs analysis and to produce an information governance strategy.

Penny decides that the target should be to get the practice to level 2 maturity across the board, and that she will use this as the target maturity for the training needs analysis.

She asks the first dentist to undertake the training needs analysis for information technology and the tool compared the input values to those required of a dentist in a practice aspiring to level 2 maturity. This led to the analysis shown in Table 64.

From your data entered, and your role, and the maturity of the practice, the model suggests you need training in:
• File management • Using a network

Table 64 First dentist IT training needs analysis

Her IM Training needs analysis resulted in the following training needs analysis report:

From your data entered, and your role, and the maturity of the practice, the model suggests you need training in:
• Clinical systems • Non-clinical systems • Data quality • Identifying information needs • Obtaining information • Clinical record keeping • Clinical decision support • Clinical communications • Clinical audit • Local Information Strategy • National Information Strategy

Table 65 First dentist IM training needs analysis

The final set of competencies concerned information governance. Again the proficiencies of the first dentist revealed major training needs compared to those needed by a dentist in a practice aspiring to improving maturity in information governance.

From your data entered, and your role, and the maturity of the practice, the model suggests you need training in:

- Knowledgeable consent
- Consent involving children
- Consent involving patients with specific needs
- Consent to use of information for research
- Consent to participation in experimental procedures
- Privacy
- Anonymity of data
- Disclosing information to immediate colleagues
- Privacy issues around sharing with other agencies
- Privacy issues for multiple purposes
- Protecting information against accidental damage
- Protecting information against unauthorised access
- Protecting information against malicious damage
- The implications of local privacy legislation
- The implications of national privacy legislation

Table 66 First dentist IG training needs analysis

Penny was able with some cajoling to persuade all of the staff to complete the three screens. She compiled the results into a training needs matrix for the practice, showing who needed training in which areas. Staff not requiring training were those who were already skilled to the required level, of that competency was not required for that role at this level. She produced one for each stream. The one for IT skills is shown in Table 67.

In those areas where most of the staff needed training she arranged workshops to address the training needs. For each individual, she drew up a training programme to address their specific issues not addressed by the communal workshops.

Technology	Dentists					Nurses					Other staff				
	1	2	3	4	5	1	2	3	4	5	Hyg	Man	Adm1	Adm2	Adm3
Personal computers & peripheral equipment					■	■		■	■	■					
Using mobile communications and computing		■	■	■	■	■	■	■	■	■	■				
File management		■	■	■	■		■		■	■	■				
Using a network		■	■	■	■	■	■	■	■	■	■	■	■	■	■
Using word processing software															
Using spreadsheet software		■	■	■	■		■	■	■	■			■	■	■
Using database software		■	■	■	■			■		■	■	■	■	■	■
Using presentation software					■			■	■	■					
Using electronic mail					■	■		■	■	■					
Using Internet / intranet					■	■		■	■	■					

Table 67 Training needs matrix for information technology for Dentown Dental Practice

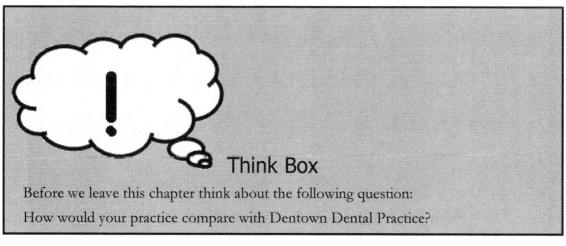

Think Box

Before we leave this chapter think about the following question:

How would your practice compare with Dentown Dental Practice?

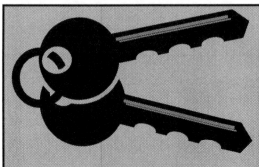

Key points from this chapter

DPIMM can facilitate and define practice improvement

The DPIMM reports identify the key tasks to be carried out in order to improve information maturity

Each level of the DPIMM requires a major change in working practices.

Chapter 12 Conclusions

By way of conclusion, here are the main points from the book, but don't forget there's lots mores useful stuff in the Appendices and on the web site.

Key points from this chapter

1. Information can improve your patient's health and your practice's wealth

2. Information technology does not deliver benefits, it delivers information which may deliver benefits with careful management

3. Governance activity must grow in sophsitication with the use of technology

4. For every risk introduced, information technology offers a better way to manage that risk

5. Computers are stupid, forgetful, literal and don't understand anything

6. On the other hand they do exactly what you tell them: they do it quickly and reliably

7. Computers can find, group and store information far more quickly than a human being

8. Because they are stupid, computers need information to be structured

9. Because they have no understanding of ambiguity, that structured information must be structured the same way every time by everybody who accesses that electronic record

10. There's lots of information out there available to your patients: they need you to help them sort the dross from the good stuff

Appendix 1   Abbreviations for dentists

Abbreviation	Country	Explanation	Further information	
			Appendix 2	Appendix 3
ABDA	Can	Alberta Dental Association		✓
ACDQ	Can	Quebec Dental Association		✓
ADA	US	American Dental Association		✓
AHIC	US	American Health Information Community (the Community)		✓
AHIMA	US	American Health Information Management Association		✓
AHIP	US	America's Health Insurance Plans		✓
AHRQ	US	Agency for Health Care Research and Quality (formerly AHCPR)		✓
AMIA	US	American Medical Informatics Association		✓
ANSI	US	American National Standards Institute		✓
ANSI ASC X12	US	American National Standards Institute Accredited Standards Committee X12.		✓
ASC	US	Accredited Standards Committee		✓
ASO	US	Administrative Services Only .		
BCBSA	US	Blue Cross and Blue Shield Association		✓
BCDA	Can	British Columbia Dental Association		✓

BCS	UK	British Computing Society		✓
BDA	UK	British Dental Association		✓
CAP	US	College of American Pathologists		✓
CDA	Can	Canadian Dental Association		✓
CfH	UK	Connecting for Health		✓
CHAMPUS	US	Civilian Health and Medical Program of the Uniformed Services		
CHIP	US	Children's Health Insurance Program/Medicare-Medicaid		
CMS	US	Centers for Medicare and Medicaid Services		
CRC	US	Code Revision Committee		✓
DBIS	US	Dental Benefit Information Service and Third Party Issues		✓
DCC	US	Data Content Committee		✓
DDPA	US	Delta Dental Plans Association		✓
DeCC	US	Dental Content Committee		✓
DHMOs	US	Dental Health Maintenance Organizations	✓	
DICOM	US	Dental Imaging and Communication in Medicine		✓
DPPC	US	Dental Practice Parameters Committee		✓
DR	US	Direct Reimbursement	✓	
DSMO	US	Designated Standards Maintenance Organization	✓	
EDI	Int'l	Electronic Data Interchange	✓	

EFMI	Int'l	European Federation of Medical Informatics		✓
EHNAC	US	Electronic Healthcare Network Accreditation Commission		✓
EHR	Int'l	Electronic Health Record	✓	
EOB	US	Explanation of Benefits	✓	
EPR	Int'l	Electronic Patient Record	✓	
ERISA	US	Employee Retirement Income Security Act of 1974	✓	
FPL	US	Federal Poverty Level .	✓	
GP	UK	General (medical) practitioner	✓	✓
HAZ	UK	Health Action Zone	✓	
HBG	UK	Health Benefit Groups	✓	
HCPAC	US	Health Care Practitioner Advisory Council	✓	
HCPCS	US	Healthcare Common Procedure Coding System	✓	
HCQA	US	Health Care Quality Alliance		✓
HEDIS	US	Health Plan Employer Data & Information Set	✓	
HHS	US	Department of Health and Human Services		✓
HIF	UK	Health Informatics Forum		✓
HIP	UK	Health Improvement Programme	✓	
HIPAA	US	Health Insurance Portability and Accountability Act of 1996	✓	
HIPDB	US	Healthcare Integrity & Protection Data Bank	✓	

HIS	UK	Health Informatics Service	✓	
HITSP	US	Healthcare Information Technology Standards Panel		✓
HL7	US	Health Level 7		✓
HRG	Int'l	Healthcare Resource Groups	✓	
HRSA	US	Health Resource & Service Administration		✓
HSC	UK	Health Service Circular	✓	
ICD	Int'l	International Classification of Disease	✓	
ICT	UK	Information and Communication Technology	✓	
IG	UK	Information Governance	✓	
IM	UK	Information Management	✓	
IM&T	UK	Information Management & Technology	✓	
IMIA	Int'l	International Medical Informatics Association		✓
ISO	US	International Organization for Standardization (ISO is the abbreviation en Francais)		✓
IT	Int'l	Information Technology	✓	
JCAHO	US	Joint Commission on the Accreditation of Healthcare Organizations		✓
LANs	Int'l	Local Area Networks	✓	
LEAT	US	Least Expensive Alternative Treatment	✓	
MDS	Int'l	Minimum Data Set	✓	

NADP	US	National Association of Dental Plans		✓
NADPF	US	National Association of Dental Plans Foundation		✓
NAIC	US	National Association of Insurance Commissioners		✓
NCPDP	US	National Council for Prescription Drug Programs		✓
NCQA	US	National Committee on Quality Assurance		✓
NDEDIC	US	National Dental Electronic Data Interchange Council		✓
NFAP	UK	National Framework for Assessing Performance	✓	
NHS	UK	National Health Service		✓
NHS IC	UK	NHS Information Centre		✓
NHSIA	UK	NHS Information Authority		✓
NICE	UK	National Institute for Clinical Excellence		✓
NPDB	US	National Practitioner Data Bank		✓
NPfIT	UK	National Programme for Information Technology	✓	
NPI	US	National Provider Identifier	✓	
NPPES	US	National Plan and Provider Enumeration System	✓	
NPRM	US	Notice of Proposed Rule Making	✓	
NSF	UK	National Service Frameworks	✓	
NUBC	US	National Uniform Billing Committee		✓
NUCC	US	National Uniform Claim Committee		✓

OCR	US	Office for Civil Rights		✓
ODA	Can	Ontario Dental Association		✓
OESS	US	Office of E-Health Standards and Services		✓
OPCS	UK	Office of Population and Census Statistics		✓
PARCA	US	Patient Access to Responsible Care Act	✓	
PCG	UK	Primary Care Groups	✓	
PCT	UK	Primary Care Trust	✓	
PHIPA	Can	Personal Health Information Protection Act	✓	
POS	US	Point of Service Plans	✓	
PRO	US	Peer Review Organizations	✓	
QA	US	Quality Assessment	✓	
QI / QIP	Int'l	Quality Improvement / Quality Improvement Program	✓	
SCDI	US	ADA Standards Committee on Dental Informatics		✓
SCHIP	US	State Children's Health Insurance Program	✓	
SDO	US	Standards Development Organization	✓	
SHA	UK	Strategic Health Authority	✓	
SMTP	Int'l	Simple Mail Transfer Protocol	✓	
SNIP	US	Strategic National Implementation Process	✓	
SNODENT	US	Systematized Nomenclature of Dentistry	✓	

SNOMED / SNOMED CT	US	Systematized Nomenclature of Medicine – Clinical Terms	✓	
STEP	UK	Standards Enforcement in Procurement	✓	
TDP / TFD	US	TRICARE Dental Program / TRICARE Family Dental Program		✓
TG	US	Task Group		
TPA	US	Third-Party Administrator	✓	
UKCHIP	UK	UK Council for Health Informatics Professions		✓
UR	US	Utilization Review	✓	
WANs	Int'l	Wide Area Networks	✓	
WEDI	US	Workgroup for Electronic Data Interchange		✓
WEDI SNIP	US	Workgroup for Electronic Data Interchange - Strategic National Implementation Process		
WG	Int'l	Work Group	✓	
WG11	US	Working Group 11: AMIA working group for dental informatics		✓
WHO	Int'l	World Health Organization		✓
X.400	Int'l	Electronic mail protocol	✓	
X12	US	ANSI Accredited Standards Committee X12		✓
X12N	US	ANSI Accredited Standards Committee X12 Insurance Subcommittee.		
XML	Int'l	Extensible Markup Language.	✓	

Notes:

1. Some of the terminology explained in Appendix 2 does not have an abbreviation so does not appear here

2. This cannot be a defintive list. It is a snapshot at December 2006, and has been edited by the author.

Appendix 2   Terminology used in this book

In a book designed to be read in different countries, particularly across the Atlantic, and across different professional groups, it is important to establish a common language. This Appendix details the terminology used in this book, and defines the way that key terms are used

Terminology	Meaning
Accredited Standards Committee	A body that develops standards in accordance with a consensus process accredited by American National Standards Institute
Administrative Services Only	A service offered by third-party payers, or third-party administrators, to manage a self-insured benefit plan on behalf of an employer group or other entity offering dental or medical benefits. In some situations a third-party payer may also provide risk-based 'stop-loss' coverage on top of the self-insured program.
Algorithm	An algorithm is a series of steps, which we can use to achieve a process. It forms the basis for most structured computer programmes. Algorithms are the subject of many weighty and incomprehensible tomes in computer science. However, the commonest type of algorithm encountered in primary healthcare is a clinical guideline, which provides a series of steps to implement a clinical procedure.
Blue Cross and Blue Shield Plans	Independent third-party payers that have agreed to provide health care benefit programs on a local basis using the Blue Cross and Blue Shield name and service marks. Each Plan may use the name and marks in specific service areas. There are inter-plan agreements that enable delivery of benefits on a national basis.
Caldicott	Review led by Dame Fiona Caldicott into the use of patient-identifiable information with recommendations on appropriate safeguards to govern access to and storage of such information.

Client Server system	A client server system is a computer system organised in two parts. The client is a local computer which sends instructions for handling files such as open, close, read, write, sort to a remote server where the data is stored. A single client may access more than one server. For a full description see the 'File Server' entry in Encyclopaedia of Computer Science, 3rd edition, Chapman & Hall, London, 1993.
Clinical Governance	A national framework through which NHS organisations are accountable for continuously improving the quality and clinical effectiveness of their services.
Clinicians	Those directly involved in the care and treatment of patients, including dentists, doctors, nurses, midwives, health visitors, pharmacists, opticians, orthoptists, chiropodists, radiographers, physiotherapists, dietitians, occupational therapists, medical laboratory scientific officers, orthotists and prosthetists, therapists, speech and language therapists, and all other healthcare professionals.
Community NHS Trusts	The NHS organisations that provide community-based services chiefly to elderly people, children and people with disabilities. Includes district nurses, health visitors, physiotherapists, occupational therapist, chiropodists.
Confidentiality	There is a legal and professional duty on dentists in all jurisdictions to keep patient data safe and prevent inappropriate access. In the UK, this is generally referred to as confidentiality, in North America as privacy
Data Accreditation Process	A systematic methodology developed in the NHS for carrying out internal reviews of the quality of data management and data outputs against clear criteria, incorporating NHS standards and recognised good practice. The achievement of standards can then be compared by external audit.
Data Content Committee	A term used in HIPAA regulations that denotes bodies whose mission includes establishing the business needs for standard transactions (electronic or paper, as applicable) within the health care community. There are three DCC's identified under HIPAA, the National Uniform Billing Committee, the National Uniform Claim Committee, and the Dental Content Committee.

Dental Health Maintenance Organizations	The equivalent of a medical Health Maintenance Organization for dentistry.
Dental Imaging and Communication in Medicine (DICOM)	An ANSI ASC whose standard for medical imaging is recognized by the ADA, and the Association is a DICOM member. The DICOM standard enables systems used in medical imaging to be interoperable.
Designated Standards Maintenance Organization	The final HIPAA rule titled "Standards for Electronic Transactions," published in the Federal Register on August 17, 2000, establishes a new category of organization, the "Designated Standard Maintenance Organization (DSMO)." Section 162.910 of this final regulation provides that the Secretary may designate as DSMOs those organizations that agree to maintain the standards adopted by the Secretary. Several Data Content Committees (DCCs) and Standard Setting Organizations (SSOs) have agreed to maintain those standards. (See DCC and SDO) (Glad that one's clear!)
Direct Reimbursement	Direct reimbursement is a self-funded program in which the individual is reimbursed based on a percentage of dollars spent for dental care provided, and which allows beneficiaries to seek treatment from the dentist of their choice.
Electronic Data Interchange	The transfer of data between different companies using networks, such as Value Added Networks (VANS) or the Internet. ANSI has approved a set of EDI standards known as the X12 standards.
Electronic Dental Record	A record containing a patient's personal details (name, date of birth etc), their diagnosis or condition, and details about the treatment/assessments undertaken by a dentist. Typically covers the episodic care provided mainly by one practice. It is a specific example of an electronic patient record, and forms part of the lifelong electronic health record
Electronic File Interchange	A standard and process for electronic bulk submission of data to facilitate mass National Provider Identifier (see NPI) enumeration.

Electronic Health Record	The term EHR is used to describe the concept of a longitudinal record of patient's health and healthcare – cradle to grave. It combines both the information about patient contacts with primary health care as well as subsets of information associated with the episodic elements of care held in EPRs.
Electronic Patient Record	A record containing a patient's personal details (name, date of birth etc), their diagnosis or condition, and details about the treatment/assessments undertaken by a clinician. Typically covers the episodic care provided mainly by one institution.
Elephant	Elephants are large grey animals found in Africa and Asia and in zoos in the rest of the world. The author alleges that many dental computer systems resemble elephants in their ability to swallow huge amounts of data, lose most of it in their gizzards, and to excrete the rest as a useless pile of dung!
Employee Retirement Income Security Act of 1974	ERISA is a federal law that sets minimum standards for most voluntarily established pension and health plans in private industry to provide protection for individuals in these plans.
Encryption	Encryption is the translation of messages into a form that is unintelligible to an outsider and is often used to improve security of information systems. The message is translated using an encryption algorithm to make it unintelligible. It can then only be decoded by use of the decryption algorithm, known as the key.
Epidemiological and Mortality Data	Health information collected to allow analysis of trends in causes of death and the pattern of illnesses.
Explanation of Benefits	A written statement to a beneficiary, from a third-party payer, after a claim has been reported, indicating the benefit/charges covered or not covered by the dental benefits plan.
Extensible Markup Language.(XML)	A flexible format designed to represent and exchange data electronically.

Federal Poverty Level	The U.S. Department of Health and Human Services (HHS) issues new Federal Poverty Guidelines every year, usually in February or March. These guidelines are commonly (yet ambiguously) referred to as the "Federal Poverty Level" (FPL), and serve as one of the indicators for determining eligibility in a wide variety of Federal and State programs.
General Practitioner (GP)	In this book, GP is taken to mean a general medical practioner in the UK sense of that word, ie the family physician with whom that patient is registered
Green Papers	Consultation papers issued by the Government providing information on current issues facing the Government and options for addressing them.
Health Action Zone (HAZ)	Designated areas in the UK where the Health Authority works in partnership with other local agencies, to specifically target local health needs.
Health Benefit Groups (HBG)	A method of linking health needs with service delivery and the expected health benefit to assist in health needs assessment and planning service delivery.
Health Care Quality Alliance	A project of the American Health Quality Association. HCQA brings together 97 national health care consumer, provider, and industry organizations dedicated to assuring that quality is the core value of the nation's health care agenda.
Health Improvement Programme	An action programme to improve health and healthcare locally and led by the Health Authority. It will involve NHS Trusts, Primary Care Groups, other primary care professionals, working in partnership with the local authority and engaging other local interests.
Health Insurance Portability and Accountability Act of 1996	US Federal legislation whose two major parts address 1) portability of health care benefits by employees, and 2) reduction in heath care administrative costs through adoption of standard electronic administrative and financial transactions, including the means to ensure the security and privacy of such information.

Health Level 7 (HL7)	HL7 is an ANSI accredited SDO that creates develops messaging standards that enable disparate healthcare applications to exchange keys sets of clinical and administrative data. The name is often used to refer the standards rather than the organisation. For example, HL7 standards are referenced in the pending HIPAA regulation concerning claim attachments.
Health Plan Employer Data & Information Set	A set of measures that are used to report the performance of health plans. The measures evaluate the organizational structure and systems of the HMO and the performance in delivering care. HEDIS was created by the National Committee for Quality Assurance (See NCQA).
Health Professional	See Clinician.
Health Service Circular (HSC)	Formal method of communication between the NHS Executive and Health Authorities, NHS Trusts and others working in the NHS.
Healthcare Common Procedure Coding System	A code set recognized for use in HIPAA standard transactions. HCPCS is divided into two principal subsystems, referred to as level I and level II. Level I is comprised of CPT (Current Procedural Terminology), a numeric coding system maintained by the American Medical Association (AMA). Level II is a standardized coding system that is used primarily to identify products, supplies, and services not included in the CPT codes. The Code on Dental Procedures and Nomenclature are listed in HCPCS as Level II "D" codes under an agreement between the ADA and CMS.
Healthcare Integrity & Protection Data Bank	The Healthcare Integrity & Protection Data Bank was set up to combat fraud and abuse in health insurance and health care delivery. HIPDB is primarily a flagging system that may serve to alert users that a comprehensive review of a practitioner's, providers, or supplier's past actions may be prudent. The data bank is intended to augment, not replace, traditional forms of review and investigation, serving as an important supplement to a careful review of a practitioner's, provider's, or supplier's past actions.
Healthcare Resource Groups (HRG)	A way of grouping the treatment of patients to allow analysis of the appropriateness of care, efficiency and effectiveness of care. Based on clinically meaningful hospital inpatient episodes and the level of resources.

ICD9/10	ICD is the commonest coding system used internationally for classifying disease for epidemiological purposes. Currently, the world is moving from ICD9 to ICD10. If Read is to be taken seriously beyond the NHS, then Read Codes must be able to be converted into ICD9 or 10 codes.
IM&T	Stands for information management and technology. Although it is commonly used in the NHS, it has to date been focused on IT rather than IM. Overseas academics tend to praise the NHS for its inclusion of IM issues. UK academics tend to ask 'Where?'
Information Governance	An umbrella term, used commonly in the UK, but less so in North America to describe the processes needed to ensure that information is processed safely, securely and in accordance with best ethical and professional practice in respect of consent, confidentiality (privacy), security and data protection.
Information Management	The way you manage your information is crucial to gaining benefits from information. It is all about making sure that you have the right information in the right format at the right time and in the right place
Information Systems Quality Assurance	The new name for systematic processes developed in the English NHS for carrying out internal reviews of the quality of data management and data outputs against clear criteria, incorporating NHS standards and recognised good practice.
Information Technology	The technology associated with information: computers, wires, keyboards, etc. Contrary to popular opinion, whilst technology can really get in the way if it's not right, it cannot deliver benefits on its own
Informed consent	Informed consent means that the patient understands the treatment and is able to make an informed decision. I think this a tall order, and tend to use the alternative term, knowledgeable consent, which appears more frequently in North America than the UK
Internet, The	The Internet is a global collection of computer networks to which anyone can gain access with a computer, a modem and a connection provided by an Internet Service Provider. The Internet is used to access the World Wide Web and for electronic mail, allowing messages to be sent across the world.

Intranets	Intranets are networks within organisations designed to provide a kind of mini-Internet for that organisation. The NHSNet is an example of an organisation wide Intranet.
Knowledgeable consent	Informed consent means that the patient is able to make a decision based upon knowledge about the benefits and risks of any procedure. The alternative term, informed consent, which appears more frequently in the UK than in North America .
Körner Data	The basic NHS data requirements devised by the Körner working party to record NHS service activity.
Least Expensive Alternative Treatment	A limitation in a dental benefit plan that will only allow benefits for the least expensive treatment. Also referred to as Least Expensive Professionally Acceptable Alternative Treatment (LEPAAT).
Local Area Networks	LANs are small-scale networks, generally within one geographical location, providing access to an information system. For example most GP patient systems operate as Local Area Networks to provide access to the system in a variety of locations throughout the surgery.
Local Authority	The body that governs local services in the UK such as education, housing and social services.
Minimum Data Set	A standard which defines the type and format of information used to record healthcare activity across a community enabling information to be shared with integrity. It provides a basic foundation on which local providers may choose to build a larger data set

MIQUEST	The MIQUEST approach and Health Query Language is used by projects in many areas of the UK National Health Service for collecting and analysing health data from fragmented incompatible systems. It was originally developed between 1992 to 1994 and 1994. The original MIQUEST project was jointly funded by the UK NHS Executive, Information Management Group and the former Northern RHA. It was established to facilitate the electronic collection of health data from commonly used general practice computer systems. To achieve this goal a structured Health Query Language (HQL) was defined. HQL is capable of expressing many current and potential requirements for data extraction from GP computer systems. As more systems are connected and standardised, the need for MIQUEST will disappear
National Health Survey of England	A national survey to provide the Department of Health with information about the health status of the national population.
National Institute for Clinical Excellence (NICE)	A new Special Health Authority to be established to promote clinical best practice.
National Plan and Provider Enumeration System	The Administrative Simplification provisions of the Health Insurance Portability and Accountability Act of 1996 (HIPAA) mandated the adoption of standard unique identifiers for health care providers, as well as the adoption of standard unique identifiers for health plans. The purpose of these provisions is to improve the efficiency and effectiveness of the electronic transmission of health information. CMS has developed the NPPES to assign these unique identifiers
National Practitioner Data Bank	The NPDB is primarily an alert or flagging system intended to facilitate a comprehensive review of health care practitioners' professional credentials. The information contained in the NPDB is intended to direct discrete inquiry into, and scrutiny of, specific areas of a practitioner's licensure, professional society memberships, medical malpractice payment history, and record of clinical privileges.

National Provider Identifier	The NPI is a unique identification number for health care providers that will be used by all health plans. Health care providers and all health plans and health care clearinghouses will use the NPIs in the administrative and financial transactions specified by HIPAA. An NPI is a 10-position numeric identifier with a check digit in the last position to help detect keying errors. The NPI contains no embedded intelligence; that is, it contains no information about the health care provider such as the type of health care provider or State where the health care provider is located.
National Service Frameworks	Evidence-based standards setting out what patients can expect to receive from the NHS in major care areas or disease groups.
National Technical Infrastructure	Encompasses a number of components that reflect national IM&T policy. For example: NHS Number, NHS Central Register, NHSnet, standard clinical codes,
Needs Assessment	The process by which a health provider uses information to judge the health of its population and then determine what services should be locally provided.
NHS 24	NHS 24 is a Scottish nurse-led telephone and internet-based information service, providing a wide range of information and advice for patients
NHS Central Register	A central database for all NHS patients. Used to monitor changes when patients move from one GP to another, and flag populations for authorised health research purposes.
NHS Clearing Service (NWCS)	A national service for ensuring that NHS contract minimum data sets are transferred to those who need them quickly and efficiently (avoiding duplication) and to support production of nationally required statistics on NHS activity.
NHS Direct	NHS Direct is an English and Welsh nurse led telephone and internet-based information service, providing a wide range of information and advice for patients
NHS Information Authority (NHSIA)	The Special Health Authority that ran information in the English NHS from 1998 to 2004
NHS Number	A unique number that identifies a patient. Everyone has been allocated a number.
NHS Strategic Tracing Service	Service provided to NHS organisations to enable them to obtain an NHS Number for individual patients.

NHS Trusts	Statutory public bodies providing NHS hospital community primary and mental health care.
NHSNet/N3	NHSNet was the name of the NHS Intranet, ie a network to connect every site in the NHS. In its original guise it never quite reached dentistry, but it is promised to do so in its new N3 guise. Not yet achieved at the end of 2006.
Notice of Proposed Rule Making	A formal process through which government regulations (eg HIPAA standard transactions) are proposed for public comment before being adopted. Such NPRM's are published in the Federal Register and these notices discuss the legislative or other rationale for the proposed rule, and specify the length of the public comment period (eg 60 days). Comments received during this period are considered and responded to when the Final Rule is published.
OPCS-4	Coding system used to record procedures carried out during delivery of healthcare.
Outcome Indicators	Measurements of the success of clinical treatment/intervention in terms of the impact on the health of the individual.
Patient Access to Responsible Care Act	PARCA imposes quality standards on managed health plans, which include: (1) requiring insurers with a 'closed network' plan to also offer a 'point of service' plan that gives enrollees access to out-of-network providers, (2) permitting enrollees to hold managed health plans accountable for plan decisions that cause them injury, (3) prohibiting managed health plans from discriminating against non-physician health professionals in plan networks based solely on their licensure, and (4) prohibiting 'gag clauses' that prevent providers from discussing with their patients the full range of available treatment options.
Peer Review Organizations	Any group of medical professionals or a health care review company that includes licensed medical professionals approved by the state insurance department to analyze the quality and appropriateness of care rendered to patients. PROs were formerly known as professional standards review organizations.

Point of Service Plans	A POS plan is a managed care program which allows subscribers to go to out of network providers. However, for this privilege, subscribers pay a higher premium and/or receive a lower reimbursement level.
Primary Care	Family health services provided by a range of practitioners including family doctors (GPs), community nurses, dentists, pharmacists, optometrists and ophthalmic medical practitioners.
Primary Care Groups	Organisations announced in 1997 which brought together family doctors and dentists, community nurses and other interests. PCGs rapidly evolved into Primary Care Trusts around 2001-02
Privacy	There is a legal and professional duty on dentists in all jurisdictions to keep patient data safe and prevent inappropriate access. In North America, this is generally referred to as privacy, in the UK as confidentiality
Quality Assessment	A methodology that obtains data that is used to evaluate the effectiveness of health care services and delivery. Surveys are one assessment tool. An objective of a quality assessment initiative is to determine what quality improvement actions may be appropriate.
Quality Improvement / Quality Improvement Program	Programs whose central goal is to maintain what is good about the existing health care system while focusing on the areas that need improvement. A QIPP is a set of related activities designed to achieve measurable improvement in processes and outcomes of care. Improvements are achieved through interventions that target health care providers, practitioners, plans, and/or beneficiaries.
Secondary Care	Specialist care, typically provided in a hospital setting or following referral from a primary or community health professional.
SMTP	SMTP is the Simple Mail Transfer Protocol, a communications protocol designed to transfer mail reliably and efficiently across networks such as the Internet.
SNOMED	SNOMED is the Systematized Nomenclature of Human and Veterinary Medicine. It is a comprehensive, multiaxial nomenclature classification work created for the indexing of the entire medical record, including signs and symptoms, diagnoses, and procedures.

Standards Development Organization	A term used in HIPAA regulations that denotes ANSI ASC's whose mission includes developing the technical solution for transmitting health care information through standard electronic transactions. There are three SSO's identified under HIPAA, Health Level 7, X12 and the National Council for Prescription Drug Programs.
Standards Enforcement in Procurement (STEP)	A methodology used to ensure the procurement of systems in line with agreed national standards.
State Children's Health Insurance Program	Dental services for the SCHIP are an optional benefit under Title XXI of the Social Security Act for all children up to age 19. However, nearly all States have opted to provide coverage for dental services. Under Title XXI, States have flexibility in targeting eligible uninsured children. States may choose to expand their Medicaid programs, design separate child health programs, or create a combination of both.
Strategic Health Authority (SHA)	Health Authorities with regional functions which oversee health care provision at a strategic level
Strategic National Implementation Process	A WEDI initiative, SNIP is a collaborative healthcare industry-wide process resulting in the implementation of standards and furthering the development and implementation of future standards. WEDI SNIP has been established to meet the immediate need to assess industry-wide HIPAA Administrative Simplification implementation readiness and to bring about the national coordination necessary for successful compliance.
Summary Personal Health Record	A short version of the primary care record containing information critical to the professions involved in caring for a patient.
Systematized Nomenclature of Dentistry	SNODENT is a large codified taxonomy of dentally related terms and descriptors that can be used to fully describe a patient's condition and dental diagnosis in an electronic medium. The development of dental diagnostic codes was initially recommended by action of the House of Delegates in Resolution 74H-1990 (Trans.1990:542). This taxonomy was based on the SNOMED architecture under an agreement between the ADA and CAP. (See SNOMED)

Systematized Nomenclature of Medicine – Clinical Terms	SNOMED / SNOMED CT is a scientifically validated clinical health care terminology and infrastructure that makes health care knowledge more usable and accessible. The SNOMED CT Core terminology provides a common language that enables a consistent way of capturing, sharing and aggregating health data across specialties and sites of care. Among the applications for SNOMED CT are electronic medical records, ICU monitoring, clinical decision support, medical research studies, clinical trials, computerized physician order entry, disease surveillance, image indexing and consumer health information services.
Teledentistry	Dental activity (including diagnosis, advice, treatment and monitoring) that normally involves a professional and a patient (or one professional and another) who are separated in space (and possibly also in time).
Telemedicine/ Telecare	Any healthcare related activity (including diagnosis, advice, treatment and monitoring) that normally involves a professional and a patient (or one professional and another) who are separated in space (and possibly also in time) and is facilitated through the use of information and communications technologies. Telemedicine is usually delivered in a hospital clinic or surgery, while telecare is delivered in the patient's home.
Third-Party Administrator	Claims payer who assumes responsibility for administering health benefit plans without assuming any financial risk. Some commercial insurance carriers and Blue Cross/Blue Shield plans also have TPA operations to accommodate self-funded employers seeking administrative services only (ASO) contracts.
TRICARE Dental Program / TRICARE Family Dental Program	The TRICARE Dental Program (TDP) is offered by the US Department of Defense (DoD) through the TRICARE Management Activity (TMA). United Concordia Companies, Inc. administers and underwrites the TDP for the TMA. The TDP is a high-quality, cost-effective dental care benefit for eligible family members of all active duty uniformed services personnel; as well members of the Selected Reserve and Individual Ready Reserve (IRR) and their eligible family members.

Utilization Review	A program for determining what health care services are covered and payable under the health plan and the extent of such coverage and payments. Such reviews come before the service (pre-determination) or after the fact (retrospective).
White Papers	Command Paper 3807, published in December 1997. Sets out the Government's programme for the modernisation of the NHS.
Wide Area Networks	WANs are large-scale networks, generally within linking different geographical locations, providing access to an information system. WANs may be made up of linked LANs. For example a PCG might establish a WAN to link the GP systems in their area. The NHSNet is an example of an information system operating across a WAN. The Internet is arguably the biggest WAN in the world.
Work Group	An acronym widely used within Standards Developing Organizations among other entities, where detailed and comprehensive work on standards and other deliverables is undertaken.
X.400	X.400 is the official international messaging/electronic email standard specified by the ITU-TS (International Telecommunications Union – Telecommunication Standard Sector). X.400 is an standard for email and electronic messaging, though less common than the more prevalent de facto email protocol, SMTP.

Appendix 3 Organisations and committees relevant to dental informatics

Many of these organisations have web sites. Look for links from the web site associated with the book.

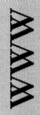

Web link

Many of these organisations have web sites. Look for links from the web site associated with the book.

I have not published URLs here because they have a nasty habit of disappearing

Organisation	Country	What they do
ADA Standards Committee on Dental Informatics	US	The ADA develops standards for dental informatics through the SCDI, an ANSI accredited SDO. SCDI's mission is: "To promote patient care and oral health through the application of information technology to dentistry's clinical and administrative operations; to develop standards, specifications, technical reports, and guidelines for: components of a computerized dental clinical workstation; electronic technologies used in dental practice; and interoperability standards for different software and hardware products which provide a seamless information exchange throughout all facets of healthcare."

Agency for Health Care Research and Quality (formerly AHCPR)	US	An agency that is part of the U.S. Department of Health and Human Services, and is the lead agency charged with supporting research designed to improve the quality of healthcare, reduce its cost, improve patient safety, decrease medical errors, and broaden access to essential services. AHRQ sponsors and conducts research that provides evidence-based information on healthcare outcomes; quality; and cost, use, and access. The information helps healthcare decision makers: patients and clinicians, health system leaders, and policymakers make more informed decisions and improve the quality of healthcare services.
Alberta Dental Association	Can	The ABDA is the professional association for the dentists in the Canadian province of Alberta
America's Health Insurance Plans	US	AHIP is the national association representing nearly 1,300 member companies providing health insurance coverage to more than 200 million Americans. These companies offer medical expense insurance, long-term care insurance, disability income insurance, dental insurance, supplemental insurance, stop-loss insurance and reinsurance to consumers, employers, and public purchasers. AHIP's goal is to provide a unified voice for the health care financing industry, to expand access to high quality, cost effective health care to all Americans, and to ensure Americans' financial security through robust insurance markets, product flexibility and innovation, and an abundance of consumer choice.
American Health Information Community	US	The Community is a federally-chartered commission and will provide input and recommendations to HHS on how to make health records digital and interoperable, and assure that the privacy and security of those records are protected, in a smooth, market-led way.
American Health Information Management Association	US	AHIMA is an association of health information management (HIM) professionals. AHIMA's members are dedicated to the management of personal health information needed to deliver quality healthcare to the public. Founded in 1928 to improve the quality of medical records, AHIMA is committed to advancing the HIM profession in an increasingly electronic and global environment through leadership in advocacy, education, certification, and lifelong learning.

American National Standards Institute	US	Founded in 1918, ANSI is a private, non-profit organization (501(c) 3) that administers and coordinates the U.S. voluntary standardization and conformity assessment system. ANSI's mission is to enhance both the global competitiveness of U.S. business and the U.S. quality of life by promoting and facilitating voluntary consensus standards and conformity assessment systems, and safeguarding their integrity
American National Standards Institute Accredited Standards Committee X12.	US	The ANSI accredited SDO that creates EDI transactions for various sectors of the business community, including Health Care. Several X12 transactions have been named as HIPAA standards. (See ANSI and X12)
Blue Cross and Blue Shield Association	US	The national association of independent BC and BS Plans that licenses use of the Blue Cross and Blue Shield names and service marks.
Blue Cross and Blue Shield Plans	US	Independent third-party payers that have agreed to provide health care benefit programs on a local basis using the Blue Cross and Blue Shield name and service marks. Each Plan may use the name and marks in specific service areas. There are inter-plan agreements that enable delivery of benefits on a national basis.
British Columbia Dental Association	Can	BCDA is the professional association for the dentists in the Canadian province of British Columbia
British Computing Society	UK	BCS is the chartered professional body with responsibility for computing and information systems and hosts many specialist groups with interests in health and medical informatics
British Dental Association	UK	BDA is the professional association for the dentists in the UK
Canadian Dental Association	Can	CDA is the federal professional association for the dentists in Canada

Centers for Medicare and Medicaid Services	US	A Federal agency within the Department of Health and Human Services (HHS) whose mission is to assure health care security for beneficiaries covered by Medicare and Medicaid programs. CMS also is the lead agency on HIPAA and health care electronic commerce activity through its Office of E-Health Standards and Services (OESS).
Code Revision Committee of the American Dental Association	US	The body responsible for determining revisions to the Code on Dental Procedures and Nomenclature. There are twelve voting members on the CRC, evenly balanced between dentistry's practitioner and payer sectors. The six ADA representatives are nominated by the Council on Dental Benefit Programs and appointed by the ADA President.
College of American Pathologists	US	The professional association that established SNOMED (See SNOMED). In November 2005 CAP's SNOMED International Division announced transfer of development, ownership and maintenance of SNOMED to an Executive Agency of the Department of Health in England, which would establish an International Standards Development Organization (SDO) for such activity. (See SNOMED)
Connecting for Health	UK	CfH is the special health authority with responsibility for delivering the English National Programme for Information Technology for the NHS
Delta Dental Plans Association	US	A not-for-profit organization, with some for-profit affiliates, that offers a nationwide system of dental health benefits for a wide range of employers.
Dental Content Committee	US	The DeCC is the deliberative body sponsored and chaired by the ADA that has been established in accordance with the administrative simplification provisions of the HIPAA to cooperate in the maintenance of the standards adopted under HIPAA. It has been named as a Designated Standards Maintenance Organization (DSMO) by the Secretary of the Department of Health and Human Services. As such, the DeCC addresses standard transaction content on behalf of the dental sector of the health care community.

Dental Practice Parameters Committee	US	The ADA began a program to develop practice parameters in 1989. During the 1993 House of Delegates, the ADA House approved a parameters development process and created the Dental Practice Parameters Committee. The DPPC has drafted proposed parameters, and at its 1994 annual session, the ADA House of Delegates approved parameters for 12 dental conditions.
Department of Health and Human Services	US	HHS is the United States government's principal agency for protecting the health of all Americans and providing essential human services, especially for those who are least able to help themselves. The Department includes more than three hundred programs covering a wide spectrum of activities. HHS-funded services are provided at the local level by state or county agencies, or through private sector grantees. The Department's programs are administered by 11 operating divisions, including eight agencies in the U.S. Public Health Service and three human services agencies. CMS is one of HHS' major agencies.
Electronic Healthcare Network Accreditation Commission	US	EHNAC was established by health care industry participants as an independent, not-for-profit accrediting body. It establishes criteria for measuring the performance of clearinghouses and value-added networks.
European Federation of Medical Informatics	Int'l	EFMI is the European Federation of national bodies responsible for medical informatics, including dental informatics
Health Care Practitioner Advisory Council	US	An advisory body established by the National Committee for Quality Assurance (See NCQA).
Health Care Quality Alliance	US	A project of the American Health Quality Association. HCQA brings together 97 national health care consumer, provider, and industry organizations dedicated to assuring that quality is the core value of the nation's health care agenda.

Health Informatics Forum	UK	The HIF is part of the BCS, and acts as an umbrella organistaion for the many specialist groups with interests in health and medical informatics
Health Level 7	US	The ANSI accredited SDO that creates develops messaging standards that enable disparate healthcare applications to exchange keys sets of clinical and administrative data. HL7 standards are referenced in the pending HIPAA regulation concerning claim attachments.
Health Resource & Service Administration	US	HRSA is an agency of the U.S. Department of Health and Human Services, and is the primary Federal agency for improving access to health care services for people who are uninsured, isolated or medically vulnerable.
Healthcare Information Technology Standards Panel	US	HITSP's mission is to serve as a cooperative partnership between the public and private sectors for the purpose of achieving a widely accepted and useful set of standards specifically to enable and support widespread interoperability among healthcare software applications, as they will interact in a local, regional and national health information network for the United States. The Panel will assist in the development of the U.S. Nationwide Health Information Network (NHIN) by addressing issues such as privacy and security within a shared healthcare information system. HITSP is sponsored by the American National Standards Institute (See ANSI).
International Medical Informatics Association	Int'l	IMIA is the global federation of national bodies responsible for medical informatics, including dental informatics
International Organization for Standardization	Int'l	ISO is a worldwide federation of national standards bodies, one in each country. The organization's objective is to promote the development of standardization and related activities in the world with a view to facilitating international exchange of goods and services, and to developing cooperation in the spheres of intellectual, scientific, technological and economic activity. The results of ISO technical work are published as International Standards.

Joint Commission on the Accreditation of Healthcare Organizations	US	The JCHAO mission is to continuously improve the safety and quality of care provided to the public through the provision of health care accreditation and related services that support performance improvement in health care organizations.
National Association of Dental Plans	US	NADP is a non-profit trade association representing the entire dental benefits industry, ie dental HMOs, dental PPOs, discount dental plans and dental indemnity products. These member dental plans provide dental benefits to 107 million of the 159 million Americans with dental benefits, ie 67% of the total dental benefits market. Member organizations include major commercial carriers, regional and single state companies, as well as companies organized as Delta and Blue Cross Blue Shield plans.
National Association of Dental Plans Foundation	US	The NADP Foundation was formed by NAPD in 1996 for charitable and educational purposes including, without limitation, to improve consumer access to affordable, quality dental care through dental benefit plans by research, education, fact finding, and the dissemination of knowledge, and to advance the state of dental health care delivery and lessen the burdens of government by formulating standards and proper courses of treatment for dental disease and conditions that can be adopted by providers, dental benefit plans, and plan fiduciaries.
National Association of Insurance Commissioners	US	The mission of the NAIC is to assist state insurance regulators, individually and collectively, in serving the public interest and achieving the following fundamental insurance regulatory goals in a responsive, efficient and cost effective manner, consistent with the wishes of its members:
National Committee on Quality Assurance	US	NCQA's mission is to improve the quality of health care. Its vision is to transform health care quality through measurement, transparency and accountability.
National Council for Prescription Drug Programs	US	NCPDP creates and promotes standards for the transfer of data to and from the pharmacy services sector of the healthcare industry. The organization seeks to support its membership in the efficient and effective development and maintainance of these standards through a consensus building process. The NCPDP retail pharmacy claim transaction (5.1) is a named HIPAA standard.

National Dental Electronic Data Interchange Council	US	NDEDIC is an organization that unites all stakeholders in the dental industry to promote electronic commerce, providing a unified forum for dental EDI. The ADA is an NDEDIC member.
National Health Service	UK	The NHS is the UK's public health service. A proportion of dentists work as independent contractors, and a smaller number are salaried employers.
National Institute for Clinical Excellence	UK	NICE are charged with deciding which treatements are deemed to clinically AND cost effective within the NHS.
National Programme for Information Technology	UK	The NPfIT is not an organisation. It is a programme run by Connecting for Health to join up all public health care in England
National Service Frameworks	UK	NSFs have been defined for the major disease groups within the UK. They define standards of care and are often used to define data collection standards to support care. As yet, there is no NSF for dentistry or oral health.
National Uniform Billing Committee	US	The NUBC was brought together by the American Hospital Association (AHA) in 1975 and it includes the participation of all the major national provider and payer organizations. This committee was formed to develop a single billing form and standard data set that could be used nationwide by institutional providers and payers for handling health care claims.
National Uniform Claim Committee	US	The NUCC is a voluntary organization that replaced the Uniform Claim Form Task Force in 1995. This committee was created to develop a standardized data set for use by the non-institutional health care community to transmit claim and encounter information to and from all third-party payers. It is chaired by the American Medical Association (AMA), with the Centers for Medicare and Medicaid Services (CMS) as a critical partner. The committee includes representation from key provider and payer organizations, as well as standards setting organizations, state and federal regulators and the National Uniform Billing Committee (NUBC). The ADA's Dental Content Committee is an NUCC member organization.

NHS Information Authority	UK	The NHSIA was responsible for information policy up to 2004
NHS Information Centre	UK	The NHS Information Centre manages various aspects of information within the NHS including many areas of standards and information governance
Office for Civil Rights	US	The Federal agency within HHS that is charged with enforcement of HIPAA privacy regulations.
Office of E-Health Standards and Services	US	The office within CMS that develops and coordinates implementation of a comprehensive e-health strategy for CMS. Coordinates and supports internal and external technical activities related to e-health services (including parts of the Health Insurance Portability and Accountability Act (HIPAA)) and ensures that individual initiatives tie to the overall agency and Federal e-health goals and strategies.
Office of Population and Census Statistics	UK	The OPCS define activity codes which are used within the UK to record activity within some health care recorsd
Ontario Dental Association	Can	ODA is the professional association for the dentists in the Canadian province of Ontario
Quebec Dental Association	Can	ACDQ is the professional association for the dentists in the Canadian province of
State Children's Health Insurance Program	US	Dental services for the SCHIP are an optional benefit under Title XXI of the Social Security Act for all children up to age 19. However, nearly all States have opted to provide coverage for dental services. Under Title XXI, States have flexibility in targeting eligible uninsured children. States may choose to expand their Medicaid programs, design separate child health programs, or create a combination of both.
UK Council for Health Informatics Professions	UK	UKCHIP is the (as yet) voluntary registration body for all professionals working in health informatics.

Workgroup for Electronic Data Interchange	US	WEDI's "core purpose" is to improve the quality of healthcare through effective and efficient information exchange and management. Its mission is to provide leadership and guidance to the healthcare industry on how to use and leverage the industry's collective knowledge, expertise and information resources to improve the quality, affordability and availability of healthcare.
Workgroup for Electronic Data Interchange - Strategic National Implementation Process	US	SNIP is a collaborative healthcare industry-wide process resulting in the implementation of standards and furthering the development and implementation of future standards. WEDI SNIP has been established to meet the immediate need to assess industry-wide HIPAA Administrative Simplification implementation readiness and to bring about the national coordination necessary for successful compliance.
World Health Organization	US	WHO is the United Nations specialized agency for health. It was established on 7 April 1948. The agency's objective, as set out in its Constitution, is the attainment by all peoples of the highest possible level of health. Health is defined in WHO's Constitution as a state of complete physical, mental and social well-being and not merely the absence of disease or infirmity.
X12 ANSI Accredited Standards Committee	US	The ANSI accredited standards committee consensus body that creates insurance EDI transaction standards for myriad sectors of the business community.
X12ANSI Accredited Standards Committee Insurance Subcommittee.	US	The ANSI accredited SDO Subcommittee that creates insurance EDI transaction standards.

Appendix 4   About the web site accompanying this book

> ## Web link
>
> This is a World Wide Web link. It refers to resources accessible via the associated Web pages which may be found at:
>
> **http://www.IT4dentists.com**

The web site associated with this book is divided into a number of sections, accessible from the left hand side of every page. On the right are more context-sensitive links, which change from page to page

You will find stuff about this book, which you will already know by this stage. You will find links to the resources referenced in the text, and to the web sites of many of the organisations listed in Appendix 3.

You will find the on-line tools for the Dental Practice Information Maturity Model, and links to active on-line resources including news feeds and discussion forums.

Appendix 5   Model answers to exercises

☑ Exercise 1 Model Answer

Patient name and address details	Patient dental details
Surname, Forename, Title DoB Sex Marital status Registered home address Previous or alternative address Telephone contact number Postcode Responsible health authority GP/Family physician	Medical, family and social history Patient contacts Symptoms and signs Dental investigations Diagnoses, sensitivities and problems Test results Acute Prescriptions Repeat Prescriptions
Financial information	Other information
Medical, family and social history Patient contacts Symptoms and signs Clinical investigations Diagnoses, sensitivities and problems Test results Prescriptions	Patient preferences Relevant miscellaneous information

☑ Exercise 2 Model Answer

Patient demographics		Patient dental details	
Information	**Tasks**	**Information**	**Tasks**
Surname, Forename, Title DoB Sex Marital status Registered home address Previous or alternative address Telephone contact number Postcode Responsible health authority GP/family physician	Healthcare Payment claims	Medical, family and social history Patient contacts Symptoms and signs Dental investigations Diagnoses, sensitivities and problems Test results	Healthcare Health Commissioning Health promotion Work closely with other agencies
How many activities?		**How good is the activity?**	
Information	**Tasks**	**Information**	**Tasks**
Patient contacts Symptoms and signs Clinical investigations Diagnoses, sensitivities and problems Test results Prescribing	Resource deployment amongst dentists Monitor performance	Patient contacts Symptoms and signs Clinical investigations Diagnoses, sensitivities and problems Test results Prescribing	Monitor performance Clinical Governance Marketing information for patients

☑ Exercise 3 Model Answer

Technical barriers	Non-computerised GPs Incompatible computer systems Lack of technical knowledge Lack of technical support
Legal barriers	Data protection legislation (UK&EU) Contractual constraints
Human barriers	Resistance to technology Resistance to change Resistance to power sharing Concerns over data quality Concerns over other threats eg computer viruses

Exercise 4 Model Answer

This is an effective solution....

Information in	Information able to searched for or sorted by
Name of practice	Name of practice
ID number of practice	ID number of practice
Address(es) of surgery	Address(es) of surgery
Telephone and fax numbers	Telephone and fax numbers
Dentist's Name	Dentist's Name
Dentist's professional ID number	Dentist's professional ID number
Dental Nurse's Name	Dental Nurse's Name
Dental Nurse's professional ID number	Dental Nurse's professional ID number
Patient title	Patient title
Patient Surname	Patient Surname
Patient Forenames	Patient Forenames
Patient identifier	Patient identifier
Date of Birth	Date of Birth
Sex	Sex
Marital status	Marital status
Payment status (Full cost/Insured with co-payment/Fully insured/Public with co-payment/Exempt)	Payment status (Full cost/Insured with co-payment/Fully insured/Public with co-payment/Exempt)
Payment history	Payment history
Registered home address	Registered home address
Previous or alternative address	Previous or alternative address
Telephone contact number	Telephone contact number
Postcode	Postcode
Responsible health authority	Responsible health authority
General Practitioner/Family Physician	General Practitioner/Family Physician
Allergies	Allergies
Date and time of consultation	Date and time of consultation
Location of consultation	Location of consultation
Medical, family and social history	Medical, family and social history
Symptoms, signs and investigations	Symptoms, signs and investigations
Treatments	Treatments
Diagnoses, sensitivities and problems	Diagnoses, sensitivities and problems
Medical prescriptions	Medical prescriptions
Interactions and contraindications	Interactions and contraindications
Doses	Doses

This is an elephant….

Information in	Information able to searched for or sorted by
Name of practice	~~Name of practice~~
ID number of practice	~~ID number of practice~~
Address(es) of surgery	~~Address(es) of surgery~~
Telephone and fax numbers	~~Telephone and fax numbers~~
Dentist's Name	~~Dentist's Name~~
Dentist's professional ID number	~~Dentist's professional ID number~~
Dental Nurse's Name	~~Dental Nurse's Name~~
Dental Nurse's professional ID number	~~Dental Nurse's professional ID number~~
Patient title	~~Patient title~~
Patient Surname	~~Patient Surname~~
Patient Forenames	~~Patient Forenames~~
Patient identifier	~~Patient identifier~~
Date of Birth	~~Date of Birth~~
Sex	~~Sex~~
Marital status	~~Marital status~~
Payment status (Full cost/Insured with co-payment/Fully insured/Public with co-payment/Exempt)	~~Payment status (Full cost/Insured with co-payment/Fully insured/Public with co-payment/Exempt)~~
Payment history	~~Payment history~~
Registered home address	~~Registered home address~~
Previous or alternative address	~~Previous or alternative address~~
Telephone contact number	~~Telephone contact number~~
Postcode	~~Postcode~~
Responsible health authority	~~Responsible health authority~~
General Practitioner/Family Physician	~~General Practitioner/Family Physician~~
Allergies	~~Allergies~~
Date and time of consultation	~~Date and time of consultation~~
Location of consultation	~~Location of consultation~~
Medical, family and social history	~~Medical, family and social history~~
Symptoms, signs and investigations	~~Symptoms, signs and investigations~~
Treatments	~~Treatments~~
Diagnoses, sensitivities and problems	~~Diagnoses, sensitivities and problems~~
Medical prescriptions	~~Medical prescriptions~~
Interactions and contraindications	~~Interactions and contraindications~~
Doses	~~Doses~~

☑ Exercise 5 Model Answer

		Instance	Implication
Strengths	Storing information	Dental records	Less space occupied
	Sorting information	Dental records	Find target groups
	Finding information	Consultation	Can find patient record
	Working quickly	Finding patient records	Can find patient record
	Doing what they are told	Reliable searching	Will find all instances
	Talking to other computers	Email file sharing	Rapid document communication
	Passing on information to other computers quickly	Email messages	Rapid communication
	Adding up and doing other sums	Accounting	Accurate and rapid
	Producing pretty graphs from numbers	Clinical Audit	Communication of data
	Sitting there and not getting impatient while waiting for the next instruction	Always available in surgery	Easier to manage than staff

Weaknesses	Not being intelligent	Literal interpretation	Need structured data
	Computers do what you say, not what you want	Literal interpretation	Staff need training
	They don't use judgement	Literal interpretation	Users need to learn new ways of working
	Bad at communicating with people	Results from searches	Need to re-present results
	Applying contextual information	Context external	If data separated from context, its meaningless
	Working with fuzzy data,	Diagnoses	User handles fuzziness
	Remembering when power is switched off	Vulnerable to data loss	Uninterruptible power supply useful
	Working the way people work	User resistance	Staff retraining needed
	Telling when people are lying	Data accuracy	Leave user in control
	Using common sense, they don't have any!	Need to check data	Leave user in control

☑Exercise 6 Model Answer

Date entered	Codes			
3rd January 2005	9082	PR1 2HE	9095(4)	
24th January 2005	9081(6)			
14th April 2005	9123 (4)			
7th June 2005	9081(6)			

☑Exercise 7 Model Answer

Barriers	Major or minor?	Motivators	Major or minor?
Lack of knowledge	Major	Facilitation of better dentistry	Major
Time to code existing records	Major	Efficiency savings	Major
Infringement on professional autonomy	Major	Help with summarising notes	Major
Inflexibility of coding schema	Minor	Training in coding and benefits	Major
Sparseness of recording	Major	Computer systems that help coding	Major
Cost of training in time and money	Major		

☑ Exercise 8 Model Answer

Information category	Retention time
Dental records	Seek legal
Demographic information	and professional
X-rays	guidance in
Financial information	your jurisdiction
Medical information	
Contact information	

☑ Exercise 9 Model Answer

Backup category	Frequency
Local incremental backup	Every day
Local complete backup	Every week
Remote complete backup	Every month

Exercise 11 Model Answer

Google.com

	Resource identified	Web address (URL)	Type
1	The Dental Informatics Online Community	www.dentalinformatics.com/	Full; requires free registration
2	Wikipedia	en.wikipedia.org/wiki/Dental_inf ormatics	Full
3	Center for Dental Informatics (CDI)	http://www.dental.pitt. edu/informatics/	Full

Google.co.uk etc.

	Resource identified	Web address (URL)	Type
1	Intute link to the DIOC	http://www.intute.ac.uk/ healthandlifesciences	Full; requires free registration
2	DHRSU	http://www.dundee.ac.uk/ /research/element6.htm	Abstract
3	GHIFT	http://www.chime.ucl.ac.uk/ resources/GHIFT/defs.html	definition

Dogpile

	Resource identified	Web address (URL)	Type
1	BUPA Promotion (!)	A Year Free at the Gym	Advertising
2	University of Michigan School of Dentistry	http://www.dent.umich.edu/ informatics/	Full
3	The Dental Informatics Online Community	www.dentalinformatics.com/	Full; requires free registration

Google Scholar

	Resource identified	Web address (URL)	Type
1	Development of standards for the design of educational software. Standards Committee for Dental Informatics.	PubMed citation at: http://www.ncbi.nlm.nih.gov/	Abstract
2	Trends in students' knowledge, opinions, and experience regarding dental informatics and computer applications	http://www.jamia.org/cgi/ content/abstract/2/6/374	Abstract
3	Dental informatics: integrating technology into the dental environment	http://portal.acm.org/	Book: citation details

PubMed

	Resource identified	Web address (URL)	Type
1	Search and selection methodology of systematic reviews in orthodontics (2000-2004).Am J Orthod Dentofacial Orthop. 2006 Aug;130(2):214-7.	PubMed citation at: http://www.ncbi.nlm.nih.gov/	Abstract
2	Accessing evidence via the Internet. Am J Orthod Dentofacial Orthop. 2006 Aug;130(2):129-30.	PubMed citation at: http://www.ncbi.nlm.nih.gov/	No abstract available.
3	Designing a framework of intelligent information processing for dentistry administration data. Int J Comput Dent. 2005 Jul;8(3):221-31.	PubMed citation at: http://www.ncbi.nlm.nih.gov/	Abstract

☑ Exercise 11 Model Answer

The following answer might be typical for a US reader, but there are analogues for UK and Canadian readers.

	Resource identified	Web address (URL)	Information provided
1	American Dental Association	http://www.ada.org	Professional information; standards information
2	American Medical Informatics Association	http://www.amia.org	Developments in informatics; conferences
3	DICOM	http://medical.nema.org/	Imaging standards
4	National Library of Medicine	http://www.nlm.gov	Literature and research material
5	Office for Civil Rights	http://www.hhs.gov/ocr/hipaa/	Privacy

Index

www.ingramcontent.com/pod-product-compliance
Lightning Source LLC
LaVergne TN
LVHW062315060326
832902LV00013B/2226